PRAISE FOR *Beyond the Label*

"With *Beyond the Label*, Dr. Christina Bjorndal brings us a brave and beautiful guidebook for regaining mental wellness. Drawing upon her own personal journey with mental illness, as well as her practice of being a Naturopathic Doctor, she offers a practical and action-oriented approach that anyone can use to initiate the self-inquiry necessary for healing. I urge you to allow these pages to speak to you, providing a new and courageous perspective that can truly set you free."
Nancy Levin, bestselling author of *Worthy*

"*Beyond the Label* is the first book to address the critical topic of mental wellness with the wide range of tactics from Naturopathic Medicine. Dr. Bjorndal has given hope through her own powerful story of recovery and the steps that made it possible."
Alan Christianson, NMD, *New York Times* bestselling author of *The Adrenal Reset Diet*

"Dr. Bjorndal's heartfelt personal journey and expert knowledge can help guide you towards light, despite the pure darkness you may be feeling. She reveals concrete steps that get to the root of the problem, instead of just covering up symptoms. Each suggestion is a step towards true healing."
Dr. Peter Bongiorno, ND, LAC, author of *Put Anxiety Behind You* and *How Come They're Happy and I'm Not?*

"*Beyond the Label* is a comprehensive resource for anyone searching within themselves for a state of mental wellness. Dr. Bjorndal's personal journey, combined with her extensive clinical experience as a naturopathic doctor, offers the reader an invaluable perspective on recovery through the mind-body-spirit connection."
Andrew Cuscianna, program director, Canadian Society for Orthomolecular Medicine

"*Beyond the Label* delivers much more than the psychobabble often found in books on mental health. Dr. Chris has created an actual blueprint for emotional healing culminating from personal anecdotal and clinical experience that reaches beyond the stigma of emotional health. Dr. Chris looks not only to discovering the root cause of mental illness and suffering, but offers practical navigation towards healing and wholeness. Finally, a truly Naturopathic perspective on mental health."
Razi Berry, publisher, *Naturopathic Doctor News & Review,* and founder, NaturalPath

"Dr. Chris goes to the very core of the beginnings of mental illness, and leaves no stone unturned to help you find the root cause of your issue. I love the way she combines science, holistic medicine and spirituality in her suggestions for therapy, holding your hand each step of the way in this beautiful guide to emotional wellness."
Dr. Ameet Aggarwal, ND, author of *Heal Your Body, Cure Your Mind*

"Dr. Bjorndal has written a very important book. It comes from her personal experience of having been diagnosed with bipolar disorder, and then treating patients with the same diagnosis. The first part walks us through her personal journey of suffering and then redemption. The second part provides hope, effective wholistic treatment paths, and opportunities for real recovery. This book should be on the shelves of every person struggling with their moods."
Dr. Jonathan Prousky, ND, author of the *Textbook of Integrative Clinical Nutrition*

Testimonials from Dr. Christina Bjorndal's patients & colleagues

"I would like first to thank you for all your help. It is always with gratitude that I think of you. You helped me realize that I needed to do much more psychological or personal work than I had realized. You helped me understand that. The good news is that I did and I achieved great results. I am doing so much better I am surprised at myself."
L.R., Vancouver, BC

"I went to Dr. Bjorndal 10 years ago because there was no place on my body that didn't hurt. My doctor said I had Fibromyalgia and suggested a treatment of anti-inflammatory drugs. Being that I wanted to be healthy I chose to seek the advice of a naturopathic doctor. Dr. Bjorndal listened to my story of life and has helped me not only to nearly eliminate the pain my body was holding as well she has enlightened me to my total body's wellness. Through such tools as morning pages, mismatched socks, supplements, detoxification programs and never letting me forget I have the power within to change any or all things that were causing my dis-ease. ... With her guidance I am looking forward to getting older and finding more freedom from the complaints that I develop when my body, mind and soul are not in agreement . . . Thank you very much for your wisdom."
W.O., Fort McMurray, AB

"I just wanted to let you know that I read your article on Eating Disorders, and I wanted to thank you for it. You were so brave! Your advice is so spot on, and I know that you are really really helping people. You have done a really good thing. Thank you for your honesty, it makes me feel that I can also be honest. Also, how you said that we are always recovering, really helped me to feel less like a failure when I have relapses in my thinking or my behaviour. You have given me renewed hope. Thank you again."
A.W.

"Dr. Chris, I can't thank you enough for all your help this past year. You have helped me overcome so many personal challenges and shown me it is possible to live the life I want and be happy and whole while doing it. Thank you for sharing your story and letting me know we're never as alone as we sometimes feel. You are an amazing person and I'm so grateful for all you do!!!!"
M.C.

"Dr. Bjorndal is a compassionate and brilliant practitioner. She is a leader in her field—mental health and women's health. I highly recommend her to anyone looking for a practitioner that has great bedside manner, and the expertise and experience to give you the tools you need to create a healthy life for you/your family. Thank you, Dr. Bjorndal!"
Dr. Monika Herwig

"You were the first person to show me kindness. You gave me a job when I had no money, listened to me without judging, and treated me with respect and compassion, which was something I had never felt. You told me things I needed to hear and nudged me forward in a very gentle way. You showed me love and gave me safety. It takes a very special kind of person to do what you do and I really admire you. Seriously, you are my hero!! I think the lesson was more about kindness than figuring out my health problems, and you were more than successful."
B.T.

"Thank you for being such a wonderful and caring human being. You are so talented and incredibly intelligent and compassionate and patient and humble. I could go on. You have helped me so much. You are definitely one of my angels. Much love to you, Christina."
J.S.

"I have been seeing Dr. Chris now for 3 years now and she has truly changed my life. I have a lot of issues including mental illness and she has been my one true hope through my journey. She speaks the truth and directly from her heart. Everything that she says to me hits home and speaks directly to my heart. She has helped me in more ways than I could ever count and I would HIGHLY recommend her to anymore."
C.K.

"The words 'Thank you' just feel so very, very inadequate for all that you've done & continue to do for me. Your knowledge, your understanding, your compassion and your never ending kindness! These are but a few of the wonderful gifts that you so generously share with those of us whom you strive to help regain our health! Thank you, thank you, thank you—I am so grateful that fate and God brought you into my life! The world is so lucky to have people like you in it! You are a Gift and a Blessing to all that know you!"
G.G.

"My wife and I met you at the end of the Brain Solutions conference. I wanted to say thanks again for your inspirational personal story and your message of hope and health."
B.R.

"I've had the pleasure of knowing Dr. Chris Bjorndal since 2001. Her passion and dedication to the art and practice of mind-body healing is inspiring. Dr. Chris applies a unique integrated orthomolecular and lifestyle medicine approach to optimize mental health. In her lectures, she speaks from the heart and courageously shares her personal healing journey to enhance the lives of others. I have no hesitation in recommending Dr. Chris for lectures and to those seeking personalized care for mental health and healing."
Dr. Sharon Gurm

"Just wanted to thank you so very much for the presentation that you gave at the Brain Solutions Conference on Sunday. I found it very insightful and, as my friend David said, 'the stuff that makes for Nobel Prize recipients—brilliance. You have an ability to take a very complex subject and make it simple and elegant.' I wholeheartedly agree. Many thanks again, with warm regards."
S.T.

"Thanks for all of the information! I'm already starting to feel better in such a short amount of time! What you have prescribed appears to be extremely effective already so thank you for everything!"
S.J.

ALSO BY DR. CHRISTINA BJORNDAL

Moving Beyond: A Journal into Self-Discovery

The Essential Diet: Eating for Mental Health

Moving Beyond Coaching Program

Mental Health Masterclass Weekend Retreat

For more information, visit naturalterrain.com

DR. CHRISTINA BJORNDAL, ND

BEYOND THE LABEL

10 Steps to Improve Your Mental Health *with* Naturopathic Medicine

NATURAL TERRAIN INC.

Natural Terrain Inc.
#200-6650 177th St. NW
Edmonton, AB T5T 4J5
naturalterrain.com

ISBN 978-0-9948020-0-2 (paperback)
ISBN 978-0-9948020-1-9 (ebook)

Produced by Page Two
www.pagetwostrategies.com
Cover and interior design by Peter Cocking

For additional information or wholesale orders, please email admin@naturalterrain.com and put "Beyond the Label" in the subject line or contact the Natural Terrain Naturopathic Clinic at 587-521-3595.

Some names and identifying details have been changed to protect the privacy of individuals.

This book is not intended as a substitute for the medical advice provided by a health care professional. The reader should regularly consult their health care provider in matters relating to his/her health and particularly with respect to any symptoms that may require diagnosis or medical attention.

17 18 19 20 21   5 4 3 2 1

This book is dedicated to all the souls who have been lost to suicide and mental illness. May we all extend our hands in grace to someone we know who is suffering.

Contents

Introduction

. . . . .

OR MANY PEOPLE, the slide into the pit of mental illness is fraught with seemingly unanswerable questions. What set it off? How could I have avoided it?

In my case, the question "Why? *Why? Why me?*" is one I have asked myself over and over again. This book is the culmination of my quest to find answers to that question—and my attempt to share these answers with readers who have similar questions. I have delved deeply into my own soul to understand the turmoil I have faced. Today, I am privileged to help many patients who struggle with anxiety, depression, eating disorders and bipolar disorders. When I work with these patients, I discuss how the following areas need to be addressed to maintain mental wellness:

1. Diet
2. Sleep
3. Exercise
4. Stress management
5. Thoughts
6. Emotions
7. Your behaviours and reactions in the world
8. Exposure to environmental toxins
9. Spirituality
10. Love and compassion for yourself and others

This book is a blueprint for the steps you can take to find balance in these 10 areas.

I will encourage you to move beyond the label (or labels) you have been given, and ask you to travel back to the centre of your being and the heart of your humanity. I want you to remember that you are more than the labels you have been assigned. Labels can serve a purpose initially, helping you to understand that there is an explanation for what you are experiencing; however, in the end, you are more than the label and can move beyond it. My hope is that you move through the stigma and shame of mental illness and find peace in mental wellness.

The ultimate lessons of this book are about how to:

- Learn to love yourself
- Find your inner voice
- Quiet the unhelpful voices of others
- Follow your path
- Live as your heart desires according to rules you define for yourself

Maybe you experience anxiety, are depressed, or struggle with your weight or an eating disorder. Maybe you have bipolar disorder, borderline personality disorder, or another mental health label. Or maybe you are just sick and tired of being tired and sick. Rest assured—you will find help in this book.

At one point, I was stressed out, depressed, anxious, obsessed with my weight, and managing it through bulimia and over-exercising. Then, after being prescribed medication to help with depression and anxiety, I had a psychotic episode and was diagnosed with bipolar disorder type 1. I thought I would never be happy. I got so low that I attempted suicide on more than one occasion. Let me tell you, there have been some very dark days.

Through all of this, I have come to learn that there are 10 key areas that need to be addressed to achieve mental wellness. I will guide you on the path to wellness, first by sharing my story and then by describing in detail the steps needed to regain mental health. My hope is that ultimately you will live a balanced life and embrace all that it can offer.

HOW TO USE THIS BOOK
....

Chapters 1 through 8 document my own struggles with mental health issues. I felt it was important to take readers through this journey of mine because only by taking it myself did I find many of the answers I am now prepared to share with you. This part of the book is very personal and will help you to understand the context for all that follows. Where I occasionally insert medical advice related to this tour through my experiences, I have titled it "Reflections from My Practice."

Chapters 9 through 21 are squarely focused on information, tips, exercises and practical suggestions that you can apply in your own life. From time to time in these chapters, I reflect back on my own journey to recount an example that helps clarify the information or advice I'm presenting. These passages are titled "Reflections from My Journey" so you can readily distinguish them from the more immediately practical information you may be looking for.

This book is designed so you can open it anywhere and start where you feel guided to start. I've repeated certain key explanations here and there so you don't need to page through the book to understand concepts that were introduced elsewhere.

Keep an eye out for the ☙ symbol, which matches important practical information with exercises you can do in your *Moving Beyond* journal to deepen your self-knowledge and further your progress.

Regaining your mental health is as simple as following the steps outlined in this book. But it is not essential that you start at Step 1. I am so excited you are holding this book in your hands! I am thrilled to be taking this journey with you. Here's to your wellness. Please know that I am always sending you healing thoughts.

DR. CHRIS

(1)

In the Beginning

. . . . .

"There are many roads to wellness. The important thing
is to pick a path and follow it wholeheartedly."
DR. CHRIS

OFTEN, IT IS HARD to pinpoint the exact moment when mental illness begins in one's life. A question we are taught to ask patients is: What was going on in your life when you were first diagnosed? I find that the answers I get to that question vary—some people remember a stressful incident, such as the death of a loved one or divorce, while others have a vague memory of their past and it all seems blurry.

When I look back on my childhood, I can remember a few incidents where I struggled with my mental health. What's difficult to differentiate is how much of that was "normal" childhood experiences (kids being kids) and how much was clinically abnormal. It didn't help that my own insecurities and anxieties seemed to be on overdrive from the moment I entered the world, given that I was adopted. I think this may have clouded everyone's judgment. As a result, most of my behaviour was chalked up to the fact that I was adopted versus the fact that I had a mental illness.

My parents decided to have one biological child and then to adopt one because my dad potentially carried the gene for Huntington's chorea, a devastating neurological disease that has been described as schizophrenia, Alzheimer's disease and Parkinson's disease all in one. My paternal grandfather had Huntington's and was institutionalized because of it. My mom lived in fear that both my dad and my brother would develop the condition and did not feel comfortable playing genetic roulette. The irony is that I, the adopted child, went on to develop a major mental illness.

My mom recounts that I was an extremely sensitive child. She remembers how her brother, my Uncle Bill, was so excited to meet me, but it took many months for me to be calm and trusting enough to be in the same room with him, let alone be held in his arms. This sensitivity has been with me my entire life. Thankfully, I have learned how to turn it into a gift rather than a curse.

Early influences

For some individuals—and often in the case of adoption—it is important to go back to when you were in utero to understand certain things about yourself. It is at this early time that neurological and emotional wiring begins; therefore, the mental and emotional state of your mother (or the person who carried you to birth, in the case of adoption or surrogacy) results in important biological imprinting. Dr. Gabor Maté discusses this in his book *In the Realm of Hungry Ghosts: Close Encounters with Addiction*. He writes:

> The important point to explore here is how stresses during pregnancy can already begin to "program" a predisposition to addiction in the developing human being. Such information places the whole issue of prenatal care in a new light and helps explain the well-known fact that adopted children are at greater risk for all kinds of problems that predispose to addictions. The biological parents of an adopted child have a major epigenetic effect on the developing fetus. Researchers from the Medical School at Hebrew University, Jerusalem, best encapsulate the conclusions of many animal and human studies:
>
> *In the past few decades it has become increasingly clear that the development and later behaviour of an immature organism is not only determined by genetic factors and the postnatal environment, but also by the maternal environment during pregnancy.*
>
> Numerous studies in both animals and human beings have found that maternal stress or anxiety during pregnancy can lead to a broad range of problems in the offspring, from infantile colic to later learning difficulties and the establishment of behavioural and emotional patterns that increase a person's predilection for addiction. Stress on the

mother would result in higher levels of cortisol reaching the baby. Elevated cortisol is harmful to important brain structures, especially during periods of rapid brain development.

Any woman who has to give up her baby for adoption is, by definition, a stressed woman. She is stressed not just because she knows she'll be separated from her baby, but primarily because if she wasn't stressed in the first place, she would never have had to consider giving up her child: the pregnancy was unwanted, or the mother was poor, single or in a bad relationship, or she was an immature teenager who conceived involuntarily, or was a drug user or was raped or confronted by some other adversity.

Any of these situations would be enough to impose tremendous stress on any person, and for many months, the developing fetus would be exposed to high cortisol levels through the placenta. A proclivity for addiction is one possible consequence.

REFLECTIONS FROM MY PRACTICE

When answering the question "Why am I the way I am?" it is important to try to identify the root causes of when things began. This is a primary tenet of naturopathic medicine.

Six principles

There are six principles that guide naturopathic doctors (NDS):

1. **Treat the cause.** NDS seek to identify and remove the underlying causes of illness, rather than to merely eliminate or suppress symptoms.

2. **First, do no harm.** Therapies should stimulate the body to heal in a gentle and effective manner, not causing unwanted side effects.

3. **Treat the whole person.** Health and disease involve a complex interaction of physical, spiritual, mental, emotional, genetic, environmental, and social factors. NDS must treat the whole person by considering all of these factors; therefore, a personalized and comprehensive approach to diagnosis and treatment is required.

4. **View yourself as a teacher.** NDS educate and encourage patients to take responsibility for their health.

5. **Use the healing power of nature**. Use natural therapies that encourage the body to heal itself.

6. **Engage in prevention**. The ultimate goal of naturopathic medicine is prevention. This is accomplished by teaching and promoting lifestyle habits that foster good health. The emphasis is on building health and using prevention as the best cure, rather than on fighting disease.

In my case, my biological mother became pregnant with me when she was 16. I don't know the circumstances surrounding my conception, except that because of her family's religion—Irish Catholic—abortion was not an option. Her parents moved her to the other side of the country—from Grand Falls, New Brunswick, to Vancouver, British Columbia—where she lived with her older sister until it was time to give birth.

Given the research cited above, it is likely that the stress my biological mother was under exposed me to cortisol, the stress hormone, at higher levels than would be experienced in planned pregnancies. As a newborn, I didn't sleep well from the beginning—something that I would make up for during many depressive episodes later in life when all I did was sleep the days and months away.

Attachment issues

The way I found out I was adopted didn't help me to attach securely to my parents. According to the attachment theory of parenting, we are all creatures of attachment, which means what we all want most is connection, attachment and relationship, whether as children or as adults. What a child wants more than anything is a connection to his or her parent, even when there is no resemblance. I feel that how I learned that I was adopted left me feeling insecure about my place in the family. Essentially, when my mom explained the word "adopted" to me, my five-year-old brain interpreted it to mean "temporary."

As adults, we tend to assume our children understand the meaning of the words we use, but in many cases, they misconstrue it. In my case, we had watched a movie at school showing animals with their offspring, and this got me thinking about where human babies came from. The advice my parents had been given by a social worker in the late 1960s was to tell me the truth about my origins whenever I eventually asked where babies came from. After watching the movie, I went home from school curious about babies and inquisitively asked how I came to be. My parents took this opportunity to explain that I was adopted. I internalized their explanation by assuming that I was only with them temporarily, and that one day, my "real" Mom would be coming to get me.

Consequently, every time the doorbell rang or my mom started talking to someone I didn't recognize at the store, I would wonder, "Is *this* the person who is coming to get me?" The years went by and no one came. I was 12 years old when I finally asked my mom if anyone was ever coming. Naturally, she was dismayed when she realized what had happened.

For me, learning that I was adopted, from the way I processed it to the negative comments from some family members to my parents—such as "blood is thicker than water"—cast a belief in me that I wasn't good enough or truly wanted. It fed my insecurities, which played themselves out on the school grounds, as I was a prime target for kids to pick on. And I did get picked on—so much so that my mom found a job at the school so I would have more support than the teachers were able to give me. Some girls in my grade four class started an "I hate Christina" club, and this devastated me. (The funny thing is, the same thing happened to my son when he was in grade two. My heart sank when he told me. But his response highlights the difference between poor self-esteem, which I had at this age, and self-confidence, which he has, because he said, "It's okay, Mom, no one joined!")

Despite my insecurities around adoption and being picked on in elementary school, there were no other traumas in my childhood. I was fortunate to be adopted into a loving family with caring parents. We moved a few times, which taught me to be resilient and accepting of others. All was well until I became a teenager and developed an eating disorder around the time my parents were getting divorced. It was then that the crack in my emotional foundation deepened.

Bulimia revealed

In my life, stress was a big problem. I had been an overachiever most of my life. I put tremendous internal pressure on myself, which stemmed from my insecurities around being adopted. I had developed a core belief that I wasn't wanted or wasn't good enough. Subconsciously, I had developed a way of operating in the world that kept these faulty core beliefs alive and true in me. I never learned to manage stress, and I kept pushing myself—top athlete and top student in high school, and Dean's list, valedictorian of my class, and athletic and academic scholarships in university. When I started working, I quickly climbed the corporate ladder, and within six years found myself in a senior management position reporting to a CEO.

REFLECTIONS FROM MY PRACTICE

Stress and the hormones that are associated with it, such as cortisol, can play a role in mental illness.

I ask all my patients how they manage their stress, and the response I often get is, "Not very well." If I had answered that same question when I was in university, I would have said that I had three primary ways of coping with stress:

- Journalling
- Exercising
- Eating—and my eating disorder: bulimia

➤ *How do you cope with stress? Use your* **Moving Beyond** *journal to write about stress and how you manage it. Are there ways you can improve? If you know what to do but don't do it, why do you think that is?*

I think an important key to my health that was overlooked by my medical doctors was the bulimic activities that I engaged in. They didn't ask the right questions, and I wasn't forthcoming in disclosing the information. So not only did I experience depression and anxiety—I was also hiding that I was bulimic.

This condition started innocently enough, when I was 15, with an offhand comment made by a friend. One day after school, I went over to my friend's house. We both gorged ourselves on junk food and then she went to the bathroom and I could hear her purging. Up until this point, it had never entered my consciousness to do such a thing. When I asked her what she was doing, she explained that it was a way to enjoy junk food but not get fat. She suggested that I might want to do this too. It was an innocent-enough remark, but it carried a lot of punch. What was she implying? Was I fat? Did I not look good?

My impressionable teenage self allowed this one-time, offhand remark to snowball into an eating disorder. The snowball wasn't rolling down a steeply pitched cliff, as it took several years for my bulimic behaviour to gain momentum and become a problem. It wasn't until I entered university a few years later that bulimia become a regular activity in my life. By this time, I was competing on the University of British Columbia (UBC) track team and striving to get accepted into the highly sought-after Faculty of Commerce. It was during my first few years of university that I resorted to bingeing and purging as my primary way of dealing with stress. I would binge on sugary foods—ice cream, cake, cookies, dough-nuts, chocolate and cupcakes—to soothe my anxiety about term papers or exams. Sugar became like a drug to me. I would desperately need to get my hands on sugar, and once I ate it, I felt a sense of relief that was quickly followed by a wave of panic and fear that I would gain weight. These fears caused me to then purge to get a further release. I spent four years being in denial about bulimia before I was finally forced to face this demon head-on in the spring of 1987.

Up until that spring, I had been using bulimia as a stress management tool. Seems crazy, right?! While my peers dealt with stress by drinking and partying, my response was bulimia. I had noticed a cycle: the more stressed I was, the more I binged, and as I ate more, I felt worse about myself, so I would then purge because I didn't want to gain weight. I didn't think I had a problem because it wasn't a daily occurrence.

It is hard for me to admit this, but often I would steal the food that I was going to binge on. However, one fateful day, I got caught shoplifting. This was extremely shameful, scary and frightening for me. I was in my car about to drive away when a young store clerk tapped on my window. I rolled down my window, and he asked me if I had shoplifted.

I didn't try to run, I didn't drive away, and I didn't back up over him. But I was stunned, shamed and shocked. The funny thing was that I was dressed in a bright neon yellow shirt—the opposite of what you would wear if you were trying not to be seen. I got out of the car and followed him back into the store. He reported me to the store manager. I have always been respectful of authority, and when the manager asked what I was doing, I burst into tears and said that I had money and could pay for everything. I explained that I stole the food because I was just going to purge it after eating, and didn't feel that I should be spending my money on something that was going to be flushed down the toilet. He told me that if I came back with one of my parents, he would not press charges.

I went home feeling terrified and frightened to death. I was overcome with fear because I was scared to tell my mom—scared of her reaction, scared that I would get a criminal record, scared that I would no longer be "perfect" in my mom's eyes, upset that I would let her down.

I called a friend who knew of my bulimic tendencies, and she said she would go to the store and pretend she was my mother. While heartwarming, this was hilarious because she was the same age as me and a different ethnicity. I thanked her, but said the store owner would see through that, and adding a lie to the mix would not get me out of the already-deep water I was in. I would just have to tell my mom the truth.

And when I did, it was fine.

She didn't scream at me or say I was a horrible daughter or that I had let her down, or question my judgment by saying, "What were you thinking?" What she did say was, "I understand. I already know. I have known for some time that you have been doing this, but in my experience, you have to wait until someone is ready to admit they have a problem before you can offer to help. Are you ready to admit you have a problem and get help?"

I answered that I was ready to admit I had a problem but that I didn't need any help.

I look back on that response and shake my head at my younger self. The resistance to "get help" is what keeps so many of us stuck in mental disease. I think for me, at that time, I really didn't believe I had an eating disorder. Even though I admitted what I had done, I was in deep denial, despite getting caught shoplifting. I viewed bulimia as a coping mechanism, not a health problem. I would simply need to find a different way to cope with the stress I was under. From that day on I made two promises to myself: 1) I would not shoplift again; and 2) I would no longer purge.

What I didn't expect, however, was the plunge into depression a few months later. Is it possible there was a connection between my bulimia and my subsequent depression?

(2)

Descent into Depression

· · · · ·

"Don't let perfection get in the way of progress."
DR. CHRIS

MY FIRST DEPRESSION began in October 1987 when I was 20 years old. The months leading up to my dive into depression and despair seemed normal—but maybe they weren't? One big change in my life was that I had stopped purging, but I still was using food and binge eating to manage my stress. It was the start of my third year at UBC. I had started the term feeling enthusiastic and optimistic about my future. Prior to attending university, I don't recall thinking that much about what it would be like. Some part of me knew it would be hard, but I certainly didn't know how hard. There would be those of us who stuck out the course, failed, took time off to work or go travelling. Or in my case—get very sick.

Feeling lost

As I entered my third year of university, many factors were at play for me. It was a trying time, and I was lost in many ways:

- I had lost my main coping skill to deal with stress, which was bulimia; however, I was still stuck in a bulimic mindset with binge tendencies.

13

- I hadn't dealt with my parents' divorce while I was in high school.
- I hadn't learned to love myself, and still believed that I was unlovable due to faulty core beliefs that stemmed from being adopted and from other events in my childhood.
- I was trying to figure out who I was, what to do with the rest of my life, what the point was of being on the planet, of being here.
- I was the classic overachiever: honour roll student (even had the highest mark in my first-year university calculus class), scholarship student (both athletic and academic), varsity track and cross-country team member. And it wasn't enough to be an athlete—I was also the team manager on top of working part-time.

Whew, it exhausts me to think about those days!

When I started university, I set out to become a lawyer. This was because in grade 10 I was interested in becoming a police officer, but it was extremely important to my parents that I go to university. We discussed why I was interested in this career, and it was decided that I would become a lawyer. I asked my dad what I should study for my undergraduate degree, and he suggested commerce. At that time, you had to complete one year of specific undergraduate courses before you could enter the Faculty of Commerce, and it was very competitive to get into the program. UBC also offered a joint Commerce-Law option, and I set my sights on that. Looking back now, I realize that the decision to study commerce was not my own. It was part of my people-pleasing tendency. I didn't have a clue what being in the Faculty of Commerce meant, what business was all about, but it seemed like the practical, logical, obvious and safe choice.

It was a steep learning curve to jump from the secure fishbowl environment of high school into the shark pit of university. When we had to choose our majors, I was feeling overwhelmed, indecisive and unsure about law school. I didn't know what else to do or what other major to choose. At the time, I couldn't identify what I was feeling—words seemed to escape me, and that feeling of general uncertainty and anxiety just kept getting stronger and stronger, to the point where I felt completely paralyzed. In fact, there was a day when I stood outside in the pouring rain without an umbrella, for what seemed like several hours, because I couldn't muster up the strength to make my legs move in any direction. I didn't know what step to take and instead remained paralyzed on the sidewalk as students moved briskly onward, passing me by. I felt like every decision I made carried so much weight. I was being crushed under the pressure of making the perfect decision.

Depression strikes

My first depression hit me like a freight train—almost like a switch. It seemed one day, I was me, and the next day, "I" was no longer there. The person I had been had disappeared behind the clouds. As the weeks wore on, I slipped further and further into the depths of depression. The only problem was that I didn't realize I was depressed and didn't have words to express what I was experiencing. I was physically, mentally and emotionally paralyzed. No one was talking about mental illness in the media at that time, and the word "depression" had never been mentioned in our household. As a result, I had no frame of reference to identify what I was going through. It was an isolating experience that left me feeling like I didn't belong in my body.

I had recently moved back home with my mom after living near the university, and had also just gone through a break-up with my boyfriend, Paul. Despite the seriousness of our relationship, I felt numb, emotionless, and I honestly didn't care whether we broke up. I sank further into depression. My mom had to help me with the basics: getting out of bed, dressing, brushing my hair and teeth, eating. I had stopped going out with my friends, stopped going to track practice, and stopped engaging with the world. When my mom went to work, I went back to bed, and I would only get up again when I heard her come home at the end of the day.

The *Diagnostic and Statistical Manual of Mental Disorders* (DSM) gives a list of nine criteria that indicate whether someone has depression (see "Reflections from My Practice" on the next page). I had all nine.

Criteria for Major Depressive Episode: DSM-5

A. Five (or more) of the following symptoms have been present during the same 2-week period and represent a change from previous functioning; at least one of the symptoms is either (1) depressed mood or (2) loss of interest in pleasure.

Note: Do not include symptoms that are clearly due to a general medical condition, or mood-incongruent delusions or hallucinations.

- Depressed mood most of the day, nearly every day, as indicated by either subjective report (e.g., feels sad or empty) or observation made by others (e.g., appears tearful). Note: In children and adolescents, can be irritable mood.

- Markedly diminished interest or pleasure in all, or almost all, activities most of the day, nearly every day (as indicated by either subjective account or observation made by others).

- Significant weight loss when not dieting or weight gain (e.g., a change of more than 5 percent of body weight in a month), or decrease or increase in appetite nearly every day. Note: In children, consider failure to make expected weight gains.

- Insomnia or hypersomnia nearly every day.

- Psychomotor agitation or retardation nearly every day (observable by others, not merely subjective feelings or restlessness or being slowed down).

- Fatigue or loss of energy nearly every day.

- Feelings of worthlessness or excessive or inappropriate guilt (which may be delusional) nearly every day (not merely self-reproach or guilt about being sick).

- Diminished ability to think or concentrate, or indecisiveness, nearly every day (either by subjective account or as observed by others).

- Recurrent thoughts of death (or just fear of dying), recurrent suicidal ideation without a specific plan, or a suicide attempt or a specific plan for committing suicide.

B. The symptoms cause clinically significant distress or impairment in social, occupational or other important areas of functioning.

C. The symptoms are not due to the direct physiological effects of substance (e.g., a drug of abuse, a medication) or a general medical condition (e.g., hypothyroidism).

O⚊ *Please take a moment to complete the checklist for yourself, and if you fit the criteria for major depressive disorder, please ensure that you let a loved one and a health care practitioner know how you are feeling.*

My university friends noticed that something was "off" with me. Some expressed their concern by sending cards and letters (this was pre-Internet, cell phone and texting days!) while others just continued on without blinking an eye. I don't blame them, as this was what business school was teaching us: that money is the epitome of success, as well as how to run a business and grow an empire. Certainly not about empathy. But two university friends who made a permanent imprint on my heart that I will never forget were Jessica and Lisa, each in her own way.

At this time, Lisa wrote me a letter:

Dear Christabelle: Please don't be sad. You are the most wonderful person: you've got so much going for you—you're incredibly intelligent, athletic, attractive, sensitive and you have a great sense of humour, which I miss. What more could you want? From what I see, you've got yourself in a dilemma where you think that every decision you make is going to influence the rest of your life, therefore, it is vital that you make the right one. But, it really doesn't matter if you realize that this is only one small stage in your life. Enjoy it! Live each day one at a time— spontaneity is fun! Make the most of what you've got today—the future will always work out—especially for someone with the qualities you have. There is a huge world out there—try to imagine you are looking down on it from space— and you will see that you are a small part of the interconnected whole. Think of yourself as part of this great world and let your problems go. Someday you will look back on this time in your life, no matter how much pain you are in now, and laugh. Watching you reminds me of a poem called "Comes the Dawn":

COMES THE DAWN
After a while you learn the subtle difference
Between holding a hand and chaining a soul.
And you learn that love doesn't mean leaning
And company doesn't mean security.
And you begin to learn that kisses aren't contracts
And presents aren't promises.
And you begin to accept your defeats
With your head up and your eyes open
With the grace of a woman, not the grief of a child.
And you learn to build all your roads on today,
Because tomorrow's ground is too uncertain for plans
And futures have a way of falling down in midflight.
After a while you learn
That even sunshine burns if you get too much.
So you plant your own garden and decorate your own soul,
Instead of waiting for someone to bring you flowers.
And you learn that you really can endure . . .
That you really are strong,
And you really do have worth.
And you learn and learn . . .
With every goodbye you learn.

Love,
Lisa

A diagnosis

Out of her concern for me, Lisa spoke to an adviser at the UBC student health clinic. She wanted to know what more she could do to help, as she knew my state was serious. I had stopped going to our track practices and was barely functioning. She was advised to make an appointment for me. I remember Lisa calling my mom (who was obviously very concerned about the changes in me) and asking her if she thought she could get me to the appointment. I had sunk very deep, and was contemplating suicide.

The thoughts were there, but I did not have a specific plan. I had feebly taken a knife to my wrists, and had thought about driving my car off a cliff or a bridge, or driving into a cement embankment. But I had not followed any of these thoughts with action. One of the biggest challenges for me when contemplating suicide was trying not to implicate anyone else in my suffering. I was trying to think of a way that would cause the least impact on anyone else, which was difficult to do.

Lisa was also terrified that I would either be upset with her for talking about me to someone else or that I wouldn't go to the appointment. Maybe on a soul level, I knew that I needed help. Even though I didn't understand or comprehend what was going on with me, there was an indifferent willingness to attend the appointment. So, I went. And it was the slow start to the unravelling of my mental anguish and the beginning of my journey on the road to mental wellness. I was diagnosed with major depression and anxiety and prescribed imipramine, a tricyclic antidepressant.

The diagnosis of depression and anxiety was a relief and a curse bundled up into the same package. I felt relief that there might be a solution, but I felt stigmatized and shamed by the mental illness labels. Even though I had been given a diagnosis, it didn't immediately lift the cloud that was hanging over me or shift the tides of self-doubt in which I was so deeply immersed. Until this point in my life, I had only learned of depression in the economic sense of the word, not the medical sense, and it was something that I didn't talk about with anyone.

Now, with the benefit of hindsight, I might refer to what happened as an "existential" crisis or "adrenal fatigue"—but I had never heard of either of those terms in 1987, let alone "depression" and "anxiety"! What I have learned since studying naturopathic medicine is that when we are under stress, our adrenal glands produce cortisol to help us deal with the stressors we are facing. When our ancestors had to run from sabre-toothed tigers, this was a useful and potentially life-saving response. More importantly, it typically did not occur daily. But today, it is as though we constantly have one foot on the accelerator; eventually, we are bound to run out of gas or burn out, with anxiety and depression as the result.

Antidepressants are designed to alleviate the symptoms of depression and anxiety by supporting neurotransmitters. However, they do little to address the root cause of one's symptoms, which may stem from hormones produced by the endocrine system. At that time in my life, I was striving for excellence in all areas: academics, sports, work and relationships. It was as if I had run out of gas because I had not learned any stress management skills. It also felt like an existential crisis because I was feeling indecisive about my career path, and I felt that if I didn't make the right decision, my life would be ruined.

REFLECTIONS FROM MY PRACTICE

Now, when I work with young adults who are struggling to decide what to do with the rest of their lives, I explain that nowhere is it written that you have to have it all figured out by the time you are 20 years old. Exploring and trying new things are how you figure out what you like and don't like. Take the pressure off yourself. Above all, don't compare yourself with others. It is important to have a direction, but don't be so rigid in your focus that you can't deviate from the plan if another direction becomes of interest.

Another UBC friend, Jessica, made an impact on me during those stressful, paralyzing, depressing dark days when I was contemplating suicide by asking me if I wanted to go for a walk. It really is remarkable how something so seemingly simple, like a going for a walk, can have a profound impact. She introduced me to places on campus that I had not taken the time to explore because I was so focused on achieving—places of beauty and art, like the Japanese gardens. These gardens are an amazing oasis amid the hustle and bustle of student life. At that time, in the depth of my despair, I didn't fully appreciate their beauty. What I did appreciate was the friendship, the connection and the fact that someone cared enough to take time out of their hectic schedule to be with me even though I couldn't form a sentence to speak or muster the strength to walk there on my own.

Jessica became my strength by taking my hand and leading me to peace. She allowed me to just be. I didn't need to talk, sound smart or impress her. She accepted me. Perhaps she recognized what I was going through and could see that I was depressed when I myself didn't know what was going on. She just sat with me in silence and showed me she cared by taking the time to be still with me. If it wasn't for friends like these (and there are many others), who knows if I would still be here today?

O⸺ *In your* **Moving Beyond** *journal, list the name of a friend you talk to on a regular basis. When was the last time you spoke? Write about how you met, what your friendship means to you, the qualities in them that you love, how they make you feel when you are around them. If you feel comfortable doing so, share this information with them.*

(3)

Ascent into Madness

"To heal the mind, you must first heal the heart."
DR. CHRIS

IT HAD BEEN three months since I started taking the antidepressant imipramine. During the first several weeks, I experienced little to no change, but then, gradually, glimpses of my old self started to appear. By early March of 1988, I noticed a considerable increase in energy, and I was sleeping less and less. By the end of the week, I had had little to no sleep for three nights. I was euphoric, fun to be with, energetic, magnetic; I had racing thoughts, rapid speech; I was full of ideas, loved life, started re-engaging with friends, went out dancing—and had no insight or self-awareness that my behaviour had become increasingly erratic.

Signs of trouble

By Friday afternoon, my mom had called my dad for help. He came over, and I spent my time showing him recent awards and papers I had written— all ego-oriented stuff that I look back on now as an attempt to gain his approval. Because he hadn't seen my depressive phase in the prior months, he also didn't see the contrast with my current behaviour, and told my mom that I seemed fine.

That night, I was going out for dinner with a friend and her older sister. We had plans to go to Seattle the next day. During dinner, my friend, who is usually the outgoing and fun-loving one, said she thought something seemed "off" with me. But I felt I was just having a good time. When I got home, I was anything but tired, despite having not slept the night before. I tried to go to sleep, but it escaped me, as it had the previous nights. I felt like I needed to talk, so I called another friend. It was late; she asked where I was, and I told her I was hiding in my closet, as I didn't want to wake up my mom. She also thought something was not right with me, but didn't know what. I talked non-stop for an hour while she listened and struggled to get a word in edgewise.

After I hung up the phone, I immediately called my ex-boyfriend, Paul, and asked him to come over. My mom heard me on the phone and asked me what I was doing. I explained that I couldn't sleep and that I had called Paul and asked him to come over. Unbeknownst to me, my mom called the emergency number that my psychiatrist had given her, and described my behaviour. She was advised to give me a warm bath and hot milk. Years later, my mom and I still laugh about this, as it seems ludicrous to suggest a bath and a snack to a person who is escalating into psychosis/mania. I suppose they thought it would be calming.

Psychosis

By the time Paul arrived, it was clear that I was ascending into madness. He was patient and kind. I hid his shoes in the washing machine. (I don't recall doing this, but I suppose on a subconscious level, I didn't want him to "leave" me. Fear of abandonment has been a deep-seated hurt that I have had to overcome in my life.) I thought I was receiving messages from the spirit of a friend's Mom and that the messenger was a cat sitting on the fence outside my bedroom window. I was certain that her mom was talking to me through the cat. I also thought that the devil would be coming to take me in the morning, and I was terrified. As I escalated into psychosis, this "god vs. devil" theme became more prominent.

Now that I work with many patients who have bipolar disorder and schizophrenia, I'm aware that the "god vs. devil" theme is commonly experienced in psychosis. I wonder if this is because Christianity has had such a strong influence on our collective consciousness, such that it has become a part of our psyche or subconscious mind. I was raised with Christian values, was always very interested in the church, Jesus and the 10 commandments. I started reading the bible in grade three after I heard someone say that it was one of the most important books ever written. Every time I have escalated into madness, this theme has been present.

Over the next few hours, as I spiralled out of control in a delusional state of psychosis, it was clear that it was beyond my mom's or Paul's ability to care for me. They tried to keep me calm and safe, but I was wild and completely out of control. I remember bouncing like a ping-pong ball between them. I would turn to Paul and ask, "Paul, do you love me?" and he would respond, "Yes, Christina, yes, I do," and I would scream that he was a liar and attack him—scratching, kicking, slapping and beating on him. I was in a mad, uncontrollable rage. There was no reasoning with me; I was completely unreachable.

I would then turn to my mom and ask her, "Mom, do you love me?" And she would respond, "Yes, yes, very much." I would get that. I trusted her. I would look deeply into her eyes and paused for a millisecond to hear, receive and take in what she had said. I would then turn back to Paul and repeat, "Paul, do you love me?" and he would respond, "Yes, Christina, yes, I do," and I would scream that he was a liar and fly into another rage.

This went on for quite some time as I went back and forth between them. It was painful for everyone. It was like I had them trapped and they couldn't leave the room. I was going back and forth between them like a wild, caged animal while, ironically, I was the one trapped in the madness of my mind.

Eventually, Paul was able to escape to call 911. He got away while my mom was attempting to calm me by holding me in her loving arms. I started to get extremely paranoid that the devil was coming to get me, and became fearful that I was going to be punished. I would not listen to my mom's voice of reason as I escalated further into a delusional state of psychosis and became increasingly lost in the madness of my mind. Perhaps a blessing of delusional psychosis is that you aren't present at all times, as you swing back and forth between madness and consciousness. As such, you cannot recall every detail later. Or maybe every detail is not recalled because it is too painful.

When the paramedics arrived, I resisted them with all my strength and power. Therefore, it took two police officers, two ambulance attendants, my mom and Paul to wrestle me into a straitjacket. I vaguely remember the ambulance ride to the hospital. The ambulance attendant reminded me of Jesus because he had a similar beard. On the one hand, I felt safe, as I thought I was being taken care of by Jesus. But I was also extremely scared because I thought that I was being driven to meet the devil. I had no idea what was happening to me. I felt out of control; everything felt surreal; all my senses were heightened, smells enhanced; I could see the dots making up the lines of lettering on the wall and the spaces between the colours. I was on sensory overload. I was in deep pain.

A new diagnosis

At the hospital, I was put in a rubber room. I exploded deeper into rage and madness and eventually was injected with haloperidol, a powerful antipsychotic medication, to calm me down. The only objects in the rubber room were a steel toilet and a mat on the floor.

For Christmas, Paul had given me a promise ring that I hadn't bothered to take off when we broke up, and in a fit of feeling betrayed I flushed the ring down the toilet. Ironically, this is something I would do again while hospitalized 20 years later, with my wedding ring. On both occasions, I didn't understand where I was. On a primal level, I felt that I had been betrayed, abandoned and deserted.

I had no concept of time while I was in isolation, but at one point, the nurse opened the door and both my parents were there. I was still in psychosis as I turned to my dad and said:

"Are you the devil?"

He responded, "No, Christina."

"Are you Jesus?"

Again, he responded, "No."

In my confused and delusional state, I turned to my mom and asked her the same questions, to which she also responded, "No." I seemed satisfied with their answers and felt somewhat calmer after being reassured by them. The door to the rubber room was shut, and I was left alone for what seemed like eternity.

Eventually, I was moved to the psychiatric ward. I was absolutely terrified to be there. The screaming and moaning that I heard from the other rooms, combined with my fear that someone was going to kill me, left me petrified. I could hardly sleep because I was afraid of the "crazy" moaning person down the hall. What if she attacks me? It never dawned on me that I was one of *them*. I was so scared and wanted to go home so badly that I lied to the psychiatrist when he came to see me in the morning. I told him I was fine. That I had slept great. I said very little, and only answered when spoken to. I "acted" normal to pass, to get discharged, and to get my "get out of jail free" card.

At that point in the episode, I wasn't fine—but I wasn't riding the wave of mania anymore. What was happening was that I now had double vision, which made it hard to look the psychiatrist in the eye, as I didn't know which of the two figures I was looking at was real. All the symptoms I was experiencing—lethargy, double vision, constipation and a flat mood/emotional numbness—were side effects of haloperidol. The prescription I left the hospital with was lithium carbonate. I was still processing and accepting the fact that I had depression and anxiety and that my eating issues were far from resolved, and now I had a new diagnosis to digest: bipolar disorder type 1.

REFLECTIONS FROM MY PRACTICE

In research, medications are studied in a random, double-blind, placebo-controlled manner. Essentially, this means they are researched in isolation from any other factors that could affect the treatment outcome. However, in clinical practice, it is more common than not for a patient to be taking more than one pharmaceutical medication. Often, they are taking a combination of two or more of the following: a sleeping pill, an antidepressant, an anti-anxiolytic, and a mood stabilizer or antipsychotic medication. This troubles me greatly, as we do not study medications and their possible long-term effects in a poly-pharmacy format. Instead, we study them over the short term in isolation. How medication was used in the research lab trials is not how it is being used by medical doctors in the field.

As a naturopathic doctor, my view of the use of both nutraceuticals and pharmaceuticals can be summed up as follows: minimum dose for maximum benefit for the shortest duration of time. The clinical challenge is that many of the nutrients required to achieve the same effectiveness as an antidepressant, for example, must be prescribed in much higher doses initially to have a result. Many times, it is easier for patients to take one 40-milligram antidepressant pill than it is to change their diet and take a variety of supplements and botanical remedies. However, the side benefits of taking a natural approach are that you will look younger and live longer.

More labels

As I learned about the condition, these were some of the other terms that flooded my mind:

- Manic depression
- Crazy person
- Paranoia
- Delusions
- Psychosis
- Locked up
- Rubber room
- Antipsychotic medications
- Mood stabilizers
- Mood disorder
- Genius
- Gifted
- Talented
- Brilliant
- Successful
- Stigma

I was discharged without any advice on how to move forward with my life or reconcile what had happened to me. That first manic episode was as shocking to me as it had been to my family and friends. We had no idea. We had no family history to go on. I had more questions than answers:

- What happened?
- How did this happen?
- Why did this happen?
- Will this happen again?
- How can I prevent this from happening again?
- Why me?

I found the new label, bipolar disorder type 1, as hard to accept as the previous labels of bulimia, depression and anxiety. I wondered if I would have lost my mind or entered a state of psychosis if I had not been taking an antidepressant in the first place. My psychiatrist offered the following explanations:

1. It is not normal to have thoughts of suicide.
2. An antidepressant will only trigger mania/psychosis if you have bipolar disorder. This suggests you have the gene for it. (I had not yet been tested for the gene; he assumed I must have it.)
3. Bipolar disorder is like being a diabetic—your body does not know how to make the neurotransmitters (in the case of depression). Therefore, like a diabetic, you will have to take medication for the rest of your life to maintain the right chemical balance in your brain.

While none of the above explanations sat right with me, who was I to question the doctor, and what did I know about brain chemistry, neurotransmitters, neuroscience or psychiatry? I had been taught that "the doctor knows best," and not to question a doctor's judgment. If the first command of a doctor is to "do no harm," then presumably the medication I was being prescribed would do more good than harm. I half-heartedly accepted the doctor's explanations, and took my medication as prescribed.

(4)

Here We Go Again, Part 1

*"Are you focusing on the possibility and promise
of your life, or the problems and pain?"*
DR. CHRIS

LOSING CONTROL IS not my idea of fun. For me, the anticipatory fear of going manic is almost as bad as actually having a psychotic episode. In my case, with each episode I've had, I have reflected and tried to learn and understand what the contributing factors were so that I can prevent it from happening again. As mentioned, my first episode was quite a shock because I had no idea that I had this predisposition in the first place. This is often the case for people who are bipolar.

The second manic episode happened shortly after the first. After being discharged from the hospital with my first episode, my mood remained in a hypomanic state over the course of the summer—that is, I was happier than my "normal" state, slightly euphoric, sleep was happening (although I needed less than usual), I had more energy, and I felt magnetic. I was dating and having a fun summer not being seriously committed to anyone.

I started my final year of university in September 1989, and by the end of October, I had slipped into another deep depression. The side effects of lithium were taking a toll on me: horrific cystic acne, shaking hands, dry/parched mouth and weight gain. The shaking in my hands was so bad that people thought I had Parkinson's disease. I remember not being able to write my final essays, as I was unable to hold a pen because my hands were shaking so badly. Instead, I dictated them to my friend. When I think about it, it amazes me that I was able to do that.

After attending a bipolar support group meeting, my mom learned of another medication that had fewer side effects. The medication, carbamazepine (brand name Tegretol), was indicated for epilepsy, but researchers had noticed during clinical trials that it seemed to have some benefits in lessening depression and stabilizing mood. In the pharmaceutical world, prescribing a drug for uses other than the one indicated is known as "off-label" use. It helps drug manufacturers find additional markets for their products. My psychiatrist agreed to switch me to this medication and at the same time started me on another tricyclic antidepressant, desipramine.

Trauma in Mexico

For the Christmas break, my mom agreed to let me go on a mountain biking trip to Cancun, Mexico, with two acquaintances, Rob and Leslie. I was depressed heading there, but the idea of travelling slightly improved my spirits. The medication had started to lift the depression, and I could function and care for myself in a basic manner.

I arrived a few days ahead of my friends, on December 24; they were scheduled to arrive two days later. I biked from the airport to the town of Cancun. (If you have ever been to Cancun, you will understand how crazy this was.) At that time, there were no shoulders on the highway for cyclists, and the drivers would barely move over to pass you. I am surprised that I survived the 12-kilometre ride to town.

When I got to town, I found a hotel to stay in until my friends arrived. I barely left my room, and spent the next few days over Christmas plunging deeper and deeper into depression. I hardly ate, as I was scared to go to restaurants or the store, didn't understand the currency, and didn't speak Spanish or recognize the food (except for tortilla chips). This trip was not getting off to the most auspicious start.

When my friends arrived, my mood improved slightly because I was with two people who thoroughly enjoyed life, and their positive energy was infectious. I was happy to follow their lead on all daily plans. We travelled to Isla Mujeres, where we were planning to spend New Year's Eve. I was sleeping well; despite the fact that my energy and activity levels were gradually increasing again, I didn't have enough insight into my condition yet to recognize the signs of advancing hypomania. In hindsight, I realized that the signals were:

- Slightly elevated energy—more than the amount I have when I am "normal." The problem was, it had been so long since I had been "normal" that I didn't recognize this as hypomania.
- Decreased desire to eat—I ended up losing 15 pounds because I was too busy to eat (and I was already underweight).
- Increased desire to exercise.
- Increased intensity and focus when listening to others.
- Increased talking—not yet to the point of where no one else could get a word in edgewise, but definitely more effervescent.
- Lots of business ideas.
- Shopping—I spent $1,000 on gifts for friends and family back home. This was out of character for me, as I am extremely financially conservative. Excessive spending is a symptom of mania that can ruin people financially or leave them bankrupt. For me, on my student budget, this level of spending was extreme. I thought I was simply being thoughtful.
- Extreme friendliness and cheerfulness—this fun-natured side of me was attracting attention from men. While I was not promiscuous, this can be a symptom of mania.

The island threw a big community party on New Year's Eve in the central square, and I participated in the fun, dancing and celebrating along with my friends. By midnight, it was clear that I was going psychotic. I ended up being separated from my travelling companions and went off with two new friends I had met on the island, Chico and Steve.

Chico lived on Isla Mujeres, and owned a local bar. Steve was visiting from England. Neither of them knew what to do with me as I escalated into madness. This episode culminated with me tearing off all my restrictive clothing, running down the street naked and being apprehended by the authorities, who threatened to put me in a military prison because they thought I was doing drugs. Thankfully, Steve was able to convince them that I needed medical attention, and I was given a bed in a three-room medical clinic. I am so grateful that my new friends were there to advocate for me, care for me and make sure that I was kept safe in the medical clinic and not put in jail. The irony of being threatened with jail while in Mexico was that 13 years later, while completing my studies in naturopathic medicine in Toronto—in my own country—I *was* put in jail during a manic episode.

It is important to understand that when someone is in the throes of psychosis, they often have very little self-awareness. I had no realization or understanding of the stress I put on my family and friends when I was unwell. From my perspective, this isn't something that is completely in my locus of control. It is not like I plan to get sick, and it is unfortunate that it happens at all to anyone. But it does. What is even more unfortunate is how people treat you when you are sick, and how little compassion there is for people with mental health issues, due to widespread lack of understanding. I was aware that my illness had negatively affected one of my travelling companions. I can imagine it is quite shocking for someone with no experience in psychosis to watch someone slip into insanity. I've been told that it is like watching someone trip out on LSD or magic mushrooms. I have never done these or any other drugs; I can only imagine that the "natural" flooding of my system by neurotransmitters is similar to the state that those who use drugs are trying to achieve. Since I was not comfortable with or accepting of mania, and thought that the mood stabilizers I was on were intended to prevent it, I was as surprised and shocked as anyone that this was happening to me again.

Over the next few days, my friends contacted my parents and psychiatrist in Canada. It was decided that my psychiatrist's intern would fly down to travel back with me on the plane, as there was some concern about me flying alone given the state I was in.

Hospitalized again

When I arrived home, I was admitted to the UBC psychiatric ward. I was there for approximately two months. Fortunately, I was able to attend my classes on a day pass, and would return to the hospital at night. I remember having a hard time when people who were admitted after me got discharged before me, especially when it didn't seem like they were better. It made me extremely frustrated to still be there. When I explained my disappointment to my nurse, he said, "You need to look at it like this. The hospital is a car garage, and we are mechanics trying to help you.

In some instances, we just don't have the parts, so the vehicle needs to be sent elsewhere. In your case, we have the parts, and you are going to leave here as a luxury vehicle." While his explanation gave me some comfort, it didn't dampen my desire to be discharged.

When I was finally discharged, I set my sights on graduation day. I was the valedictorian of my graduating class. While my parents were extremely proud of my accomplishments, I was still stuck in the stigma and shame of having a mental illness. Here is the speech I gave:

Upon graduation, the question that can be heard ringing through the halls is "WHAT AM I GOING TO DO NOW?" For many it is an uneasy sensation, similar to what one feels when they discover that an hour's preparation or cramming before a midterm exam isn't quite enough.

After five years of commerce, I truly feel that we are now ready to face the challenges that lie before us, each of us having suffered through and completed our degrees. From our many experiences at UBC, we should cherish the good aspects, such as friendship. I think the most rewarding experience of our university careers has been the friendships that have developed over the last five years. Such friendships have instilled feelings of togetherness and sharing, the sharing of ideas, feelings and ambitions. These are true friendships that will remain with you a lifetime, they are to be treasured and valued like no other.

We should also learn from the bad, that is, don't let your failures pull you down, but may they provide you with an incentive to work harder and continue to strive toward the most prestigious of achievements. In anything you set out to do, do not accept mediocrity. Advancement cannot occur in the world if individuals simply desire sufficiency or adequacy, rather than excellence.

I think now, more than ever before, we have realized we must work hard for what we want. We must take responsibility for our lives and persevere. At UBC, we've learned not to accept indifferent efforts from ourselves. Each one of us has a strong feature or talent that distinguishes us from one another and this talent has hopefully been strengthened during the past half-decade. In whatever you aspire to become, develop your talent to the fullest and use it to your advantage. Goals are dreams and wishes that are not easily reached. You have to work hard to obtain them, never knowing when or where you will reach your goal. BUT KEEP TRYING!!! Do not give up hope, and most of all

never stop believing in yourself. For within you, there is someone special, someone wonderful and successful. No matter what you achieve,
as long as you want it and it makes you happy, you are a success.

You must employ your privileged position as university graduates as
a positive influence as you venture into the work force. It is imperative
to realize that we, as the youth of today, and as the contributors of our
society tomorrow, will have the capacity and, moreover, the responsibility to steer society in the direction in which we wish it to go. We must
remember that the experience and knowledge we have accumulated
over the past 17 years represents only the start of our real education. To
quote Winston Churchill: "This is not the end. It is not even the beginning of the end. But it is, perhaps, the end of the beginning." Good luck
to you all and thank you!

A job and a move

I was extremely fortunate to have received a job offer at the beginning
of the school year to work at HSBC Canada as a commercial lender, and
I moved to Calgary, Alberta, in September 1990 to start my career in
banking. At the start of my banking career, the advice I had been given by
my psychiatrist was to not disclose my mental health condition to anyone.
Business can be cutthroat, and he didn't want it used against me. I felt
like I had to keep my diagnosis a secret due to a general lack of understanding and acceptance regarding mental health conditions.

(5)

A Decade of Depression

"Are you thinking about the past or worrying about the future?
Remember to ask yourself where you are living in your mind,
because you only have the present moment."

DR. CHRIS

THE 1990S WERE anything but stable for me, despite being free of psychosis and mania. During that time, I was riddled with anxiety, depression and major stress. There can be so much emotional angst during a person's twenties anyway, and I was still trying to figure out what I wanted to do with the rest of my life. I felt like I had to get that right and couldn't make a mistake. I felt caught between the pressure of the 1950s stay-at-home Mom and the Gloria Steinem feminists of the 1970s. There was a part of me that wanted to get married, have five children and "settle down"; however, I had no prospects, as my dad liked to point out. What was I supposed to do in the meantime?

My mom had never had the opportunity to finish her university studies. She was always encouraging me to be my own person, go to school and follow my heart. The problem was that I lived to please my parents. I felt caught between them after their divorce, and didn't really know anymore what *I* wanted, let alone who *I* was or what *I* stood for.

I loved working at the bank... at first. The excitement of moving away from home was empowering. But after a short period in Calgary, I was transferred to Nanaimo, British Columbia. There, I was met with a patriarchal mentality and "old-school" management style that was not supportive of female commercial lenders. In fact, I was the first female commercial lender at that branch. Historically in the banking industry, commercial lending was a male domain and women were relegated to customer service roles. With the difficult branch environment, lack of support from management and lack of community, I noticed my mood shifting. I began to slip into another depression.

And so went the 1990s, which for me were characterized by oscillating between climbing out of depression and slipping back into it. I flirted with suicidal thoughts throughout these years, and they finally became prominent in the beginning of 1994. By this time, I had been transferred two more times with the bank, ending up in Burnaby, British Columbia, at the beginning of 1994. Over the course of the next several months, a deep depression set in.

Surviving suicide

On June 9, 1994, I attempted suicide. The months leading up to this attempt were very dark. Six months prior, I had been promoted as a commercial lender, but unbeknownst to me, the branch manager had "fixed" the commercial portfolios so that the one I managed had all the problem accounts while the other portfolio manager handled all the A+ accounts. I was spending countless hours at work, feeling like I was drowning in it and in completely over my head. It wasn't a good sign that I knew the janitor by his first name, as I often worked until 10 p.m.

REFLECTIONS FROM MY PRACTICE
....

A common question asked of someone who is depressed is "Why are you depressed?"

With each depressive episode I have had, I have reflected on this question and asked myself, "What happened? Why did I get depressed? What did I do wrong?"—as though it were completely in my locus of control to regulate my mood by magically turning a switch on or off. I have come to learn that this is not a question you ask someone who is depressed. Most people don't "choose" to be depressed—or do we? Maybe on a subconscious level, we do because, deep down, I know that I didn't love myself or accept myself. Was that the real cause of all my pain?

So, what exactly happened that night, and why? At that time in my life, I had expected the promotion and transfer to Burnaby to be positive, as I was now closer to my family and friends. As with any episode, it was multifactorial:

1. I didn't foresee how much I would miss the wonderful friends and colleagues in my previous community. Because I was now working so much, I found it hard to make time for my family and friends in Burnaby. As a result, I became socially isolated.

2. I didn't realize the impact the real estate market would have on me. I moved from a two-bedroom, 980-square-foot apartment to a one-bedroom, 675-square-foot apartment for two-and-a-half times the price. I didn't foresee the anxiety I would feel from being "tied down" by the weight of my mortgage payments. It physically crushed my chest, making it difficult to breathe at times. I bought just before the leaky condo bubble burst in Vancouver, and watched in dismay as my property value plummeted. Because of this financial obligation, I felt chained to a job I was growing to dislike more and more each day—like an animal trapped in a cage with no options for escape.

3. I was naive about business politics and didn't anticipate the lack of support I would receive at the new branch. I had no idea that my portfolio could be composed primarily of bad debt accounts.

4. Because the distribution of my portfolio was unequal, I worked 10- to 14-hour days from January to June. The important things I usually did to maintain mental wellness—like exercise and eat properly—were neglected. As such, my exercise regime became compromised, and my vegetarian diet consisted of frozen foods and canned soup. Hardly healthy or nutritious.

5. My self-confidence steadily declined as I felt I was in over my head at work and too proud to admit it or ask for help. The seeds of self-doubt

grew into uncontrollable weeds that I could no longer pluck from my consciousness. My judgment was clouded by negative self-talk that was defeatist and seemed to grow louder as the months wore on. I got so tired of listening to the constant barrage of verbal abuse I directed at myself that eventually I believed the only way to be free of it was to commit suicide. Then and only then would there be silence.

I was seeing my psychiatrist regularly. As in previous depressive episodes, it often took several months of sliding deeper into the pit of depression before I could muster up the strength to say I needed more help. Many times, words were not needed as my psychiatrist could determine from my affect that something was not right. For example:

- I would not talk during our sessions, as I had nothing to say.
- The blank look of hopelessness in my eyes spoke volumes.
- The visible weight loss I experienced was evidence that I had lost the desire to eat or nurture myself.
- Other signs of depression included the endless hours I would spend in bed not wanting to face the day, my work responsibilities, or my life; or the social isolation that I fell into, as I no longer found joy in being around my friends or family, since it was an effort to "put on a happy face." Also, I no longer had the desire to exercise. I felt a lot of shame and guilt around the self-deprecating thoughts I had, and would not admit that I was suicidal unless my psychiatrist directly asked the questions "Do you have thoughts of suicide? Do you have a plan?"

I was prescribed a new antidepressant, Zoloft, in February 1994. During my previous depressive episodes in the early 1990s, I had been prescribed Prozac; however, I was assured that Zoloft was "new and improved." It was later discovered that there is a connection between suicide and Zoloft, and that "suicidal ideation, thoughts, and behaviour—collectively termed as suicidality, and suicidal acts have long been linked to antidepressant usage. Selective serotonin reuptake inhibitors [SSRIs], including sertraline (Zoloft), are believed to increase suicidality risks."

Searching for an explanation

Ultimately, I think it was a combination of the various stresses in my life (i.e., moving, new job, intense portfolio, financial stress, lack of socialization, poor diet, no exercise, poor self-esteem, etc.) that resulted in the events of June 9, 1994. What I remember the most are the thoughts that plagued me. The self-critical thoughts that repeatedly told me that I was worthless, I was no good, that no one cared about me, that I might as well kill myself, etc. If my voice of reason piped up with a rebuttal, such as "That is not true, you have worth," then the voice of doubt would quickly put me in my place, countering with comments like, "You are such a chicken, you can't even kill yourself. You aren't even good at *that*!"

The tug of war between these two sides of me was exhausting. I had such a hard time turning off those thoughts that after six months of being terrorized by them, I decided the only way to stop them was to end my life. On June 5, 1994, I wrote this in my journal:

> Well, it's been two months since I've written and things haven't been going that great. I'm still very unhappy with life, my job, etc., and I can't seem to figure out what is the problem. I am definitely depressed. I've been to my psychiatrist, who put me on an antidepressant (Zoloft), which has helped a bit, but not a lot! I have to try and figure out why/ what it is that's making me feel this way. Is it work? Do you like what you do? Can you even answer that question? I'm not thrilled with the branch manager or the other commercial lender. I don't really trust them, especially when they go behind my back and authorize commercial deals that I've just declined without even explaining it to me so I can learn.
>
> Is it your love life? What love life! Well, not really because I'm not ready for a serious relationship right now. I'm not interested in physical contact. The companionship would be welcomed, but it's not really that.
>
> What about the fact that you've been wanting to take your life! You have to make a decision either way—you make your life better by changing what is bothering you—or you give up. To give up is a cop out, I suppose, but it seems like a pretty good option at times. Over the past eight weeks you've been trying to think of other career opportunities— cop, teacher, your own business or Outward Bound, but nothing has really happened— you haven't come to any conclusions except you want to quit your job. But why?! Do you hate banking? What would align better with your values and interests—health, nutrition, helping others? I wish I never decided to do a commerce degree and go into business/ banking. Well, no decisions have come now with this writing. I may or may not talk to you later depending on how things unfold. Don't compare yourself to others; just do the best you can do. Maybe you should

go in and talk to the branch manager— tell him how much you dislike your position right now. Maybe I am in over my head—ask him what he thinks I should do?

And that was it. I never talked to anyone about how I was feeling. I never mentioned that the thoughts of self-doubt had been plaguing me for six months. Thoughts that constantly told me: I wasn't good enough, I was stupid, I was a loser, I was not worth the breath I was breathing, and so on.

Four days later, I tried to kill myself by drinking antifreeze. (Note: If you are depressed and reading this, please do not try this. Please reach out for help by calling a loved one, a suicide hotline in your area or 911 in North America.) As I set the glass down, a sense of panic washed over me. *OMG, what have I done. Do I want to do this? Yes, yes,* answered the voice. *I am tired. I have had enough of this life. I am done. It will all be over in the morning.*

I fell asleep hoping that I would never wake up again, that my life would be over and I would finally find out the truth about heaven, God, white lights, the meaning of life and "the afterlife."

The next morning, I was barely conscious. I tried to get out of bed, but I had lost all motor function in my lower limbs. I flopped out of bed onto the carpet and dragged myself through the closet into the bathroom. I somehow made it onto the toilet, but I fell off. I could have easily smashed my head on the tub or the counter, but I didn't. My head felt like someone was trying to split it in half with a sledge hammer. I didn't remember what I had done the night before. I was extremely nauseous and felt like I was going to vomit. I hung my head over the toilet and was still thinking that I could get myself to work on time. And then, I passed out.

That morning, I was supposed to be at a breakfast meeting with my boss. When I didn't show up, my boss called the customer service manager, Mandy, at the branch to see if I had forgotten about the meeting and had instead gone to the office. Alarm bells went off when they realized that I wasn't there. Mandy called my dad, who was unavailable, as he was in a meeting. She then called my mom. She was out of the country at the time, visiting my brother in Japan, but my stepfather happened to be home, as he had a dentist appointment (normally he would not have been there to answer the phone). He knew I had been depressed, so he raced over to my apartment.

He made his way into the building and found me barely breathing. He called 911; I was rushed to the hospital. Again, I was blessed, as the emergency room doctor had special training and knew to insert a dialysis line in the larger femoral vein (versus the smaller subclavian vein, as was standard practice). I later found out that this is one of the reasons why my life was spared. By using the larger vein, my blood could be cleared of the poison faster. This meant that there was less poison available to damage my vital organs. I remained in a coma for a few days in the intensive care unit. When I regained consciousness, I was extremely nauseous and unwell. Think of the worst flu symptoms you have ever had and then multiply them exponentially. I had tubes coming out of me everywhere and felt extremely depressed and disappointed that I was still on the planet.

I was put on dialysis, as my kidneys were not functioning. I was told that I would need a kidney transplant if they did not recover. I can tell you that I was certainly not impressed when I realized that not only had I been unsuccessful in my suicide attempt but also I now might be "handicapped" for the rest of my life. I even remember when the ER doctor came to check on me, I honestly had a hard time looking at her as I wished she hadn't used "heroic measures" to save me. I was as far from gratitude as I could possibly be, and couldn't even muster up the grace to thank her.

A new beginning

While I was in recovery, my friend Lisa gave me a book to read by Marianne Williamson called *A Return to Love*. There was a section in the book on surrender:

> Surrender means the decision to stop fighting the world, and to start loving it instead. It is a gentle liberation from pain. But liberation isn't about breaking out of anything; it's a gentle melting into who we really are. We let down our armour, and discover the strength of our Christ self. We are simply asked to shift focus and to take on a more gentle perception. That's all God needs. Just one sincere surrendered moment, when love matters more than anything, and we know that nothing else really matters at all. What He gives us in return for our openness to Him, is an outpouring of His power from deep within us. We are given His power to share with the world, to heal all wounds, awaken all hearts.

I didn't grow up in a family that expressed love verbally. I don't think I've ever heard my dad say, "I love you." And I doubted his love, partly because I doubted that I was lovable. I looked at being adopted as a negative thing. I was Unwanted. Unloved. Discarded. That was the story I told myself repeatedly. This has since shifted for me, but at this time in my life, I was still stuck in that negativity, with those beliefs guiding me. When I was in recovery from suicide, my moment of surrender came when I was at my dad's. I knelt on the bedroom floor, my head resting in my dad's lap as he sat on the bed. I surrendered to God. I remember saying, "I didn't do this to be a gimp for the rest of my life. Please, God. Please. Help me." I didn't want to remain on dialysis, nor did I want to have a kidney transplant. I prayed for my kidneys to heal. I sobbed.

My dad sat in silence and stroked my hair. He allowed me to be. He didn't try to change the moment with words. He didn't shame me or say, "How could you have been so stupid?" He just allowed the space of silence to be filled with his loving presence. After several minutes of listening to me sob heavily, he said, "It will be okay."

And so it was. A few weeks later, my kidneys made a physical recovery, and I celebrated the fact that I could urinate again. Never in my wildest dreams could I have imagined this being something I would want to celebrate! My nephrologist said I was a walking miracle, and that given the amount of poison I had consumed, I really should not be here.

Maybe I am a walking miracle. All I know is that in that moment on my knees, I had reached my lowest point. My heart was finally open and I was as vulnerable and raw emotionally as I have ever been (other than when I have been in a manic state). Even though my kidneys had made a physical recovery, I still had a lot of work to do mentally, emotionally and spiritually.

REFLECTIONS FROM MY PRACTICE

While recovering in the hospital, I read about a research project that involved two groups of AIDS patients. One group accepted their condition and had a strong support system. The other didn't accept their condition, lived in shame because of it, were shunned from their communities and did not have any family support. Researchers compared the outcomes of these two groups.

Not surprisingly, the positive group lived longer lives and had better prognoses as well as less severe symptoms and fewer complications from their health condition.

What dawned on me at that point in my recovery was that I had not accepted myself. I was living in shame because of my mental illness, and still did not want anyone to know about it. I had also been told by my psychiatrist to not disclose my mental health history to anyone at work. This kept me in the closet and stuck in shame. Today, I advise patients to be open about their condition, at least with trusted friends and family members, so they can accept themselves, avoid or reduce any shame, and have better outcomes overall.

The sole reason I became a naturopathic doctor was that when I was struggling with my illness, there weren't many natural mental health experts in practice. Now, many years later, I have made it my life's work to help those who are struggling with their mental health using natural therapies. This book will be your guide along the road to recovery.

After reading *A Return to Love*, I began to think about healing. How do I recover? How do I learn to love myself? Is there another way to feel, other than depressed and anxious or in fear of mania? Slowly, very slowly, a crack of light began to shine through my broken heart. I figured that perhaps God wanted me here and it wasn't my time. Since reading that book, I have made accepting myself and my diagnosis my number one priority. It has become my primary objective and goal in life to find natural ways to manage the mental illnesses that I have had to overcome: bulimia, anxiety, depression and bipolar disorder type 1.

Return to work

I was terrified to return to work. Thankfully, when I went back, there was a new branch manager and I was able to make a new start. One of the first things I did was find out the hours I was supposed to be working and stick to that schedule. I tried to have a better work-life balance than I'd had the previous year, and I got back to a regular exercise program. A friend had once advised me to get to work before my boss and leave after him to convey the impression that I was hard-working. I now think that is unhelpful and ridiculous advice; productivity is not about how many hours you sit in your office, but, rather, what you do while you're there. After my suicide attempt, I decided that I was going to "work to live," not live to work.

I also planned a vacation to Australia in early 1995. While I was travelling, I couldn't deny that my current career was not what I wanted to do for the rest of my life; however, I was unsure what else I wanted to do. When I returned from my trip, I applied to fill a maternity leave position for nine months. I decided that I would use that time to figure out what it was I really wanted to do with my life. Unfortunately, instead of doing that, I kept getting promoted, and I continued to climb the corporate ladder for the next five years. After the maternity leave position ended, I was asked to work on a special project with an executive from HSBC Group head office in London, UK. The bank was looking to acquire an investment management firm in Canada, and I was tasked with working on the merger and acquisition of the firm, M.K. Wong & Associates. When this was completed, I ended up in a senior management position reporting directly to the CEO of HSBC Asset Management (Canada) Ltd. I had a secure job, a wonderful team of co-workers, and a bright future ahead.

But there was always this tiny whisper from my heart nudging me to make a change. Despite these whispers, the decision to make a career change was clouded in self-doubt. I had done lots of personal growth work since 1994, but despite my best efforts, I still had dips of depression and suicide attempts requiring hospitalization. I was still taking far too much medication to manage my mind, and I was still in search of answers.

(6)

The Big Decision

"The goal is to move from self-improvement or self-judgment
to self-acceptance and self-love."
DR. CHRIS

IT TOOK ME many years to muster the courage to leave my secure job
at HSBC. I knew I wanted to leave or make a change several years earlier, but I didn't know to what. I took a long, hard look at my life and
didn't like what I saw. I was alone, I hated myself, and I was still battling
depression, anxiety, binge eating and body image issues. I was terrified
that someone would find out that I was bipolar and my reputation and
credibility would be stripped from me. I was battling sexism and inequal-
ity in the workplace and then if I did do well at work, I perceived that the
people I beat out didn't like me because I got the job. Everywhere I turned
I felt unsupported.

In researching this book, I found this journal entry from when I was
getting up the courage to leave my job:

> Why do you want to leave your job so badly? Well, I'm not interested.
> It's not really where I want to be. People have always said, "Oh, you're
> so smart" and I took that to mean that I better do something great with
> my life. But working at HSBC isn't it, even though I have a great job and
> report to a CEO. I'd like the time to figure out what I want to do. Go back
> to kindergarten if I have to, and start all over. I'm feeling a pit in my

47

stomach because this is very scary, but at the same time I am excited. Now maybe some doors will open. I'd also like to take some time to visit with Granny and Mom a little more—maybe do more for Mom—not sure what I can do, but helping her in the garden might be a good start. So, how are you feeling? What thoughts are going through your head? I must admit I have doubts, there are definitely doubts. I have that pit in my stomach, sort of a nauseous feeling. I am thinking about what my mom said: "Don't look for happiness in your job because not many people find it . . ." And when I hear that statement I wonder why not me? Why can't I love what I do? Why can't I find something I enjoy more, be it for less money, and be happier? It is interesting how exhausted I am all the time. What Cheryl [one of my best friends] said made sense, that perhaps I am exhausted because I am using all my energy up on an issue that is emotionally draining. For me, it is work and my relationship. [At the time, I had been dating Steve for two years.] Okay, now I am having tightness in my chest. Be present with that, Christina. What is that all about? Maybe do the "I'll-be-happy-when" exercise. For me, it's "I'll be happy when":

1. I leave my job at HSBC.
2. I find some other work that interests me.
3. I work at a low-pressure job, like operating a ski hill chair.
4. I become a teacher.
5. I have my own business.
6. I move in with my partner.
7. I become a naturopathic or orthomolecular doctor.
8. I write my book.
9. I become an advocate for something I believe in.
10. I can be myself.
11. I can know myself.
12. I can be true to myself.
13. I can be true to others.
14. I am not exhausted all the time.
15. My health is better.
16. I acknowledge my feelings.
17. I listen to my feelings.
18. I listen to my inner spirit.
19. I learn from the inside out.

20. I live from the inside out.
21. I am free of the chains that bind me—what are those chains?
    - Work
    - Weight
22. I am helping others.
23. When I am in control.
24. When I call the shots for me.
25. When I know what I want.
26. When I know who I am, what I stand for and what I am interested in.
27. When I know where I want to live.

I'll be happy when all this is done.

Now I feel like you should keep working until you have a plan. Is that your voice or your parents? I think it might be my parents. What would you say to a friend? I would say "You'll know when it is right . . . only you can decide."

○━ *Journal homework: Do you have a list of conditions that you need to satisfy before you can be happy? In your* **Moving Beyond** *journal, write about your "I'll-be-happy-when" list. Remember that happiness is not something you wait for. It is available to you now.*

The search to change my career led me to explore the idea of developing an organic baby formula with two friends: Lisa (mentioned earlier) and Janet. While doing the research for that project, I attended the Canadian Health Food Association's tradeshow and learned about a public talk on mental health. At that lecture, I listened to Dr. Abram Hoffer, who was a nutritionally oriented (orthomolecular) psychiatrist. He talked about using vitamins and minerals to help people regain their mental health. I left the event filled with optimism that there was another way to help manage my mental health conditions without the use of pharmaceutical medication.

The turning point

I am where I am today because of Dr. Hoffer, as well as the work of my other health care professionals. My initial understanding and awareness that nutrients play a role in mental health was due to Dr. Hoffer. Prior to becoming his patient, only my naturopathic doctor had tried to teach me that what I was eating would affect my mood and how I felt. I had been a vegetarian, but I was more like a "carboterian," as I was not a "good" vegetarian. I also had been bulimic, so my nutritional foundation had a deep crack in it. While I was no longer a vegetarian or bulimic, I still had a poor diet. After my university running days, I became a triathlete and had a few nutritional deficiencies: iron, vitamin B12, zinc, omega 3s and tryptophan.

Dr. Hoffer prescribed essential nutrients that my body required in order to make the "feel-good" neurotransmitter serotonin. I was suffering with anxiety and depression when I started his protocol in October 1999, and within a few weeks, I felt them lift. After 15 years, I wondered if I was finally free from the roller-coaster ride of depression, anxiety (general and social), bipolar disorder type 1 and bulimia.

When I felt better, I was able to take stock of my life. I hadn't been able to do this before because I was so stuck in the stigma and cloud of the mental labels I had been given that I couldn't see beyond them. When the clouds lifted, I began to experience joy, happiness, a sense of calmness, peace and comfort. I was then able to take a look at my life, my values and my direction. It was after listening to Cheryl Richardson, a life coach and author, being interviewed by Oprah Winfrey that my life changed with one question. During the episode, she encouraged the audience and viewers to contemplate the following: "If money didn't matter, what would you be doing with your life?"

I sat with that question, and what came up for me was, "become a naturopathic or orthomolecular doctor and help people regain their mental well-being, as I have." My next thought was, "Are you crazy?! You can't quit your job! You can't leave the secure position you have at HSBC!" Thankfully, I was able to take a deep breath and not be swayed by self-doubt, fears and insecurities. This was a change that my heart, had desired since I encountered my first depression in university. The only difference was that I was learning to listen to the voice of my heart, or intuition, versus the voice of fear from my mind. In February 2000, after deliberating for several years, I resigned from my position at HSBC and went back to school (first high school, then UBC) to get the science prerequisites that I would need to get into naturopathic medical school. I was 33 years of age.

When I went to see Dr. Hoffer, he was in his eighties, and I knew that he wasn't going to be able to help people forever. Today, the Mood

Disorders Society of Canada reports that one in five Canadians will experience a mental illness in their lifetime. That is far too many, as far as I am concerned. When Robin Williams committed suicide, it sparked much discussion on the topic of mental health. When I was first diagnosed in the late 1980s, there was no conversation going on. *None.* While I am happy to see the shift to having an open dialogue over the past 30 years, I think we need to move from talking about it to doing something about it. What are we doing to enact change? It has been reported that by 2030 one person will commit suicide every second somewhere in the world. We have a silent epidemic going on, and we all need to be a part of the solution. I would like to change this statistic. This book is my part in offering a solution.

OPEN. SEE. FEEL. BELIEVE. CHANGE.

Open your mind
Open your eyes
Open your heart
To the belief that change can happen

See in your mind
See in your eyes
See in your heart
The change happening

Feel through your mind
Feel through your eyes
Feel through your heart
A change in belief

Open. See. Feel. Believe. Change.

A poem I wrote after learning of Robin Williams's death

(7)

Here We Go Again, Part 2

*"If the past leads to painful memories—then it is best
to stay in the present moment."*

DR. CHRIS

AFTER FEELING SO much better after starting Dr. Hoffer's protocol, I began to wonder if I was "cured." Maybe the doctors had
been wrong and I wasn't bipolar. After all, I had never had a psychotic episode naturally. I had always been on some form of psychotropic
medication when it happened. When I had questioned my psychiatrist
about this, he told me that a "normal" person would never experience
mania on medication; only those with the genetic tendency for mania
would. Since I am adopted, I didn't have a family history to verify the
validity of that statement. This left a suspicion in the back of my mind, or
maybe it was a refusal to accept the label. I continued to take my medication, along with the supplements, for fear of getting sick again. It had now
been a decade since I had been manic, and I began to question whether
it would ever happen again.

Well, it did. While the allure of mania has been described as addictive,
for me, it is a state that I have feared and have tried desperately to keep
hidden. The irony is that mania is impossible to hide. It begs to be seen.
And while it can be fun to be in a hypomanic state leading up to a full-
blown psychotic event, it usually comes with an inevitable downswing
into depression as the pendulum swings the other way. Mania is the yang
to the yin of depression.

Back to school—and another manic episode

The first two months after leaving HSBC were good. Initially, I was excited about my studies. Slowly, though, my insecurities got the better of me. I started to feel overwhelmed about the length of time it was going to take to become an ND. Would I even be accepted into the program? Would I pass once I got there? I began exploring other career options that would guarantee me a paycheque sooner rather than later, such as teaching or becoming an RCMP officer or city police officer. I thought maybe I could use my business skills in a transferable position in the health field. Or maybe Steve would propose and I could get married and become a mom.

Partly because of the struggles my boyfriend and I were having in our relationship, we attended a personal growth course called "The Art of Happiness." Leading up to the course, I had been sleeping well, but after the first night, I only got a few hours of sleep. During the course, there was some intense emotional work, and I found that I was very triggered by the energy of the other group members.

I escalated into mania on the third day of the course and ended up jumping into the Fraser River. In hindsight, the course organizer should have called an ambulance for me, but instead, she sent me in a cab to St. Paul's Hospital, where I was left—in a state of psychosis—to check myself in to the hospital. This was not going very well for me, as I was losing my mind and I am sure I looked like a street person in the baggy clothes I had been given to wear after changing out of my wet clothes.

I ended up calling Lisa, who contacted Janet (we all had been working on the organic baby formula project). Janet was a resident in emergency medicine at the hospital. Lisa had already played an instrumental role in supporting me with my health challenges, and I now believe that Janet also was in my life for the same reason. Ultimately, we all helped each other move our lives in alignment with our spiritual paths, as we were all searching for courage to make big changes in our lives but didn't know how.

Here is an account of the experience, written from Janet's perspective:

The phone rang as I was washing dishes on a cloudy Sunday afternoon. "Janet, Chris just called me from emergency. She said to call you and then hung up. Something's wrong." I was at the hospital in minutes, where I found my friend at triage crying. She clung to me, and as she spoke, things became clear. I recognized the pressured speech, the loud voice, and the hyperactive behaviour. As an emergency resident, I had encountered it many times. However, this time it was my friend, and the experience changed forever the way that I view psychiatric patients and the medical system as a whole.

Before I continue, let me say that this is not a criticism of the dedicated staff at this hospital and other emergency rooms across the country. We all do the best we can in the crunch that is acute medicine. However, I hope that my experience may help people step outside of "the box," if just for a moment. The box is our comfort zone. Inside it we exist in a state of clinical detachment, using characteristic language and attitudes with respect to patients; both are defence mechanisms that enable us to do this challenging work. For example, I was shocked to hear my friend referred to as "the bipolar," forgetting my own frequent similar references to patients. I honestly can't remember referring to a patient by their name in the emergency department. Unfortunately, I will probably step back into that familiar box in a matter of days or hours, but wanted to record this experience at a time when I was able to view things from an eye-opening perspective.

Before I arrived, Chris had been told there were no psychiatric beds available, and that there would be none available for days. She possessed enough insight to know that she needed inpatient treatment, but was rather dramatic about it because of her condition. As well, before arriving at the hospital, she had jumped into a river and lost some of her clothes. She came across as an angry street person, perhaps even strung out on coke. Not the vivacious, inspiring young professional who until recently had been a high-level manager in an international corporation.

I don't mean to imply that her "status" should entitle her to more respect or better care. However, I'm sure many in the waiting room would have been surprised by the information. Alone, afraid, and paranoid, there was no way she could check herself in to triage without some help, and she wasn't getting it. Luckily, I arrived just as she was considering going back out onto the street. The last time she was this sick, she made a serious suicide attempt and ended up in the ICU.

As soon as I had calmed her down, I started to grasp at strings. I knew the on-duty emergency physician, who made some calls and informed me that there were no psych beds in the city, and that I should try to get her admitted. Meanwhile, Chris had been insisting loudly that she needed her psychiatrist's number, saying that he wanted her to call him at home. Of course, we'd never dream of giving a physician's home number to any patient, much less a psychotic screaming one. I was skeptical myself, but used my hospital badge to get into the nursing station, where I asked the unit clerk for the psychiatrist's number. It wasn't listed, so I picked up a phone, identified myself as a resident to the switchboard, and got it.

I then called the psychiatrist, who confirmed that he had given her his number and said that he would contact the on-call psychiatrist, making her an urgent priority for admission. When I told the triage clerk, he repeated that there were no beds and that she would likely not be admitted, as there were eight people in line ahead of her. He was quite unfriendly, even though he knew that I worked there. He was probably justifiably annoyed that in the midst of a backed emergency department, I was using my connections to push a friend through. However, I persisted, and got her checked in.

When I went to visit her the next day, she was ensconced in her corner of the acute psychiatric unit, surrounded by flowers and friends. All, including Chris, were thankful that she was alive and safe. In addition, I was feeling some disconcerting emotions. Seeing a friend in a psychotic state had been profound. Despite her "crazy" condition, she had still been very much herself. Beneath the bizarre behaviour and delusions, it was actually quite easy to find the person I knew. With a chill of awareness, I had to acknowledge that I had regarded psychotic patients as being somehow not of themselves. I hadn't considered that the healthy person might be preserved within, aware at some level of what was happening. I don't mean to be putting forward a theory on psychosis or mania; I am only trying to express what I discovered about myself. I'm sad to say that I had not been seeing or treating these patients as people.

Furthermore, I had discovered what it was like to be on the outside, desperate to get care for a loved one and running into one brick wall after another. "Sorry, you'll have to wait" and "there are no beds," echo in hospitals across our country every day. I'm used to saying these words, not hearing them. I chose to ignore these words because of my position, which I'm sure many would criticize me for. When you're desperate you'll try anything. My heart goes out to those who don't have anything to try.

Thus ends my story, with a happy ending for my friend and a number of lessons for me. Hopefully I won't forget them; that was part of my motivation for putting this to paper. If you even gain a fraction of the awareness that I achieved from writing this, it will make this effort worthwhile to me.

This piece was submitted for publication in the *Canadian Medical Association journal* but was rejected. I am extremely grateful for how my friend was able to help me, that she was home to answer the phone, and for the risks she took to get me safely admitted.

This was my third manic episode while on prescription medications. I began to wonder what the point was of taking a mood-stabilizing medication if it couldn't prevent mania. My psychiatrist explained that there isn't a medication strong enough that you can take on a daily basis to override mania and still function in some capacity. Trying to prevent mania is analogous to trying to stop a volcano from erupting. While the supplement regime had been effective at stabilizing my mood from a depression and anxiety perspective, I questioned the need for pharmaceutical medication that wasn't doing its job in that area, nor with preventing mania. I began to search for answers on how to prevent mania from ever happening again.

While I was recovering in the hospital, I read about a job opening at *Alive Magazine* for a marketing manager. I applied for the position, attended the interview while on a day pass from the hospital, and got the job. I planned to start the job two weeks after I was to be discharged from the hospital. I remember that I was nervous in the interview that my hospital bracelet might slip under the cuff of my shirt and expose me.

While I was happy to be working again, the job was short-lived, as the owner of the company was very short-tempered. He never seemed satisfied, and I found it a difficult environment to work in. It is very unlike me to quit anything, as I grew up with the belief that once you take something on, you should see it through. But sometimes I think quitting can be a source of strength. It allows you to recognize what is not serving you and to realize that you no longer have to remain stuck in a situation that isn't best for you. Quitting can open the door to freedom and allow you to pursue other paths that may be better suited to you.

However, the timing of leaving my job was not ideal. My boyfriend and I had broken up a few weeks prior, and Christmas was two weeks away. I am certain my mom was concerned I would plunge into another depression. Thankfully, I didn't. Instead, I went back to my original plan to become a naturopathic doctor, and began pursuing my dream of completing an Ironman event, which I did in 2001.

Three more manic episodes

Since being diagnosed with bipolar disorder type 1 in 1988, I have had a total of six manic episodes, three of which I describe in more detail below.

2003

Around this time, my then-boyfriend (now husband), Michael, was graduating from naturopathic medical school in Toronto, and his mom, dad and sister were flying in from the Yukon for his graduation. I have always struggled with being accepted and wanting people to like me, and, true to form, I had been putting a tremendous amount of pressure on myself to ensure his family would accept me. Despite these pressures, by all accounts, I was doing "well" in the weeks leading up to their arrival. Unfortunately, the day they arrived, the volcano erupted.

The night before this episode, I'd had less sleep than usual, but nothing that I felt was unmanageable. I had planned a run with my friend Jeannie, and we set off as usual on what should have been a routine course. But halfway through the run, I went psychotic: One minute we were running and having an intelligent conversation, and like a switch had been flicked, I flipped into mania. I suddenly stopped in my tracks, got down on my knees, and began laughing hysterically while speaking in an incoherent, bizarre manner. This was quite alarming for Jeannie, another naturopathic medical student, as I hadn't told her about my "secret." She knew that something was terribly wrong with me but didn't know what. Fortunately, she was able to guide me back home. When we got back to my house, she stayed with me until Michael arrived.

He found me naked in the corner of my bedroom, curled in the fetal position, rocking back and forth. Jeannie explained what had happened, and Michael called 911 and put some clothes on me. The police showed up quickly, but they didn't believe I had a serious mental health condition. They accused me of using drugs. I didn't want to go anywhere with them, and was waiting for the ambulance to arrive—but it didn't seem to be coming.

Michael tried to explain that this was a medical matter and that I needed to be taken care of by paramedics, but his pleas fell on deaf ears. The police showed no compassion to either of us. They did not try to reason with me but instead barged forward on the faulty assumption that I was strung out on drugs. As I resisted going with them, one police officer stood between Michael and me while the other dragged me kicking and screaming up the stairs to the main floor of the condo. The police officer told Michael in a very unsympathetic tone that he needed to stay back and out of the way because this was now a police matter. When the police officer dragged me to the top of the stairs, my screams turned primal, as he had me on the ground with his knee digging into my back, twisting my arm painfully behind it. At that point, the police officer accused me of assaulting him, forcefully handcuffed me and shoved me into the back of the police car. They whisked me away without advising Michael where they were taking me.

I was taken to Sunnybrook Health Sciences Centre to be admitted. But when we arrived, I refused admittance. The intake person said there was nothing she could do for me if I didn't want to be admitted. The police put me back into the car and tried another hospital, but I refused admittance again. Judging that this would be a pattern, but not wanting to take me home either, they drove me to the downtown Toronto police station instead and put me behind bars in a holding cell. Meanwhile, Michael was frantically trying to find out where they had taken and me. By the time he arrived at Sunnybrook, we had left.

When Michael arrived and found out that I had refused admittance, he took off on a wild goose chase to find me. It took persistence, patience and detective work to find out where I was.

The night I spent in the holding cell was an unreal experience. I couldn't understand why the police officer had cut the elastic out of my pants or whose clothes I was wearing. I was not given any medication or sedatives. I was left with my own delusional, psychotic mind to try to make sense of where I was and what was happening to me. I was frightened and lost, felt powerless, and was not being listened to. I was unwell and in need of love, care and compassion that I wasn't getting in the police environment.

Going manic is an experience that is profoundly difficult to describe to someone who has not experienced it. To date, I have not seen it depicted properly in any Hollywood movie. But as my friend wrote in her article—and as I can personally attest—even in the midst of psychosis, the "normal" person is still there behind the delusions; there are moments of clarity and normalcy as you oscillate in and out of madness.

Although I didn't fully understand what was happening to me, I knew I didn't belong in a jail cell. In the morning, I had to appear before a judge. Michael worked with the Crown attorney to convince the judge that I needed medical attention. This was the day of his convocation and graduation. His family had flown in to be part of it. And Michael missed it. He missed all of it. His father understood that he was doing what a real doctor should—he was caring for me.

After I was finally allowed to leave the police station, I was taken by the police to Toronto General Hospital, and this time, I agreed to be admitted. But it still wasn't going to be smooth sailing. The handcuffs were replaced with a straitjacket. I was left strapped to the bed in the middle of the emergency admitting area, as there were no beds available in the emergency room or the psychiatric ward. I was not treated with dignity, like a human being should be—more like a wild animal. When the MD came near me to inject me with haloperidol (an antipsychotic), I flew into uncontrollable convulsions, which made it extremely difficult for him to inject me despite the fact that I was tied down.

On top of that, the severe acute respiratory syndrome (SARS) epidemic was raging at the time, so I was treated by MDs who seemed to be wearing space suits, which was disorienting in my state. Also, due to SARS, Michael was not allowed to visit me because he had already set foot in the lobby of Sunnybrook, and the health system in Toronto was working in overdrive at the time to try to prevent the spread of SARS between hospitals. If he had stayed outside at Sunnybrook, he would have been able to visit me at Toronto General, but because he had set one foot past the emergency room doors, he was deemed at risk for SARS and was denied access to the next hospital he visited.

Upon being discharged from the hospital, I had to appear in court to avoid a criminal record because the police officer had brought an assault charge against me. I don't recall assaulting anyone, but I do recall being treated with unnecessary physical force by the police officer. To this day, an area of my neck and back remains traumatized from being forced into the police car against my will. Thankfully, when I appeared before the judge, he was very empathetic and compassionate, and threw the charge out. Upon recounting this episode, I now regret that I did not file a formal complaint with the Toronto Police Service for the way I had been treated.

Although this is perhaps a topic for another book, my treatment during manic episodes has led me to believe that police officers in most cities need much more training than they seem to be getting in how to respond properly to people who are mentally ill. I have nothing but praise for the other first responders who have had to deal with me over the years (firefighters, paramedics), but the police have been the opposite of compassionate, understanding and patient. This needs to change.

And it is happening slowly, with joint mobile program initiatives in place in many major Canadian cities (e.g., Montreal, Halifax, Toronto, Hamilton, Edmonton and Vancouver). This requires a mental health worker to respond to crisis calls with the police. Initial reviews suggest there are many benefits to these co-response programs. It is important to emphasize that these initiatives need to be integrated into a broader strategic approach for all police agencies.

2006

When Michael was at naturopathic school (1999 to 2003), he befriended a woman in his class named Stella. For two years, he fostered their friendship, but deep down he had hoped their relationship would develop into something more. He had finally given up on that, and about a year later, he met me. Michael and I had been dating for a few months when, one day, he came to my dorm room laughing so hard he was crying. He said, "All this time, I thought there was something wrong with me, and now I've found out why Stella was never interested in me—it's because she's a lesbian! She plays for the other team!"

We ended up becoming very good friends with Stella and her partner, Catherine. In fact, Catherine was my student clinician at the Robert Schad Naturopathic Clinic, and both Stella and Catherine had been involved in helping Michael during my previous manic episode in 2003. They had provided him with homeopathic remedies to help my recovery.

After we all graduated from naturopathic medical school (Michael and Stella in 2003, Catherine in 2004, and I in 2005), we all got busy setting up our practices and moving on with our lives.

After he had graduated, Michael moved back to the Yukon (Whitehorse), as he wanted to serve the First Nations communities there and show his gratitude to the band that had supported him financially through naturopathic medical school. Stella and Catherine ended up moving to Winnipeg, since that was where Catherine was born and raised. And when I graduated, I moved from Toronto to Vancouver, where I began sorting through everything I had put in storage during the years I'd been studying. I then moved everything to Whitehorse to be with Michael.

Shortly after I arrived in Whitehorse, Michael was offered the opportunity to take over a colleague's practice in Fort McMurray, Alberta. As his heart was in the Yukon, we decided to work half of each month in Fort McMurray and the other half in Whitehorse. During the summer months, we commuted between the cities—a 26-hour drive! During those long road trips, we planned our wedding, and Michael would quiz me for my upcoming board exams.

After we got married, Catherine contacted me to apologize for not coming to our wedding. It turned out that Stella and Catherine also got married in October 2005. Up until this time, however, Stella had kept her relationship with Catherine private, as she came from a strict Greek Orthodox background and wanted to "spare" her mother the challenge of processing the news that she was a lesbian. Shortly after their wedding, it became clear to Catherine that Stella was not herself. Stella escalated into hypomania in early November 2005. Their relationship spun out of control directly because of this. Stella became resistant to any help from Catherine, and the situation became extremely stressful. Catherine made a heart-wrenching decision to leave the relationship at the end of December 2005 due to the intensity of living with someone who was mentally unwell but unwilling to accept help.

Stella did not react well to this decision, and continued to verbally abuse Catherine for months until Catherine ultimately decided to cut off all communication with her. This break in communication was short-lived, as Catherine cared deeply for Stella and knew she needed help. The escalation into hypomania had come at a time of increased stress for Stella, as her mother had passed away.

After the break-up, Stella moved back to Toronto while Catherine remained in Winnipeg. It was an emotionally upsetting time for both. I had been in communication with Catherine, but we were unable to get in touch with Stella. While talking to Catherine and a few other friends, I learned that Stella's behaviour was becoming increasingly erratic. As news about Stella came to us from various sources, we tried to contact her, but our attempts were met with silence and dead ends. Catherine became increasingly worried about Stella, but didn't know what to do or how she could help, given the emotional and geographical distance between them.

Meanwhile, I had found out I was pregnant; we would be expecting our first child in May 2006. As winter approached, driving back and forth between the two cities become increasingly unrealistic, so we decided to make the commitment to Fort McMurray and moved there in November 2005. While it was a busy and exciting time, it was also very stressful. The beginning of 2006 started off as a whirlwind: I wrote my board exams in February, received my licence in April, and six weeks later gave birth to our son and went on maternity leave. Four weeks after that, I turned 40.

While I was happy to become a mother, I had yet to solidify myself in my new career as a naturopathic doctor, and I felt overwhelmed. I'd had little time to practise before going on an unpaid maternity leave. I felt stressed on many fronts: starting a new career and business, moving, being newly married, giving birth, being a new mom and enduring sleepless nights with a newborn and no family support, experiencing financial stress and the isolation of living in a Northern community. Unbeknownst to me, these were setting me up for the perfect storm. Mania loomed on the horizon.

A few months later, in August 2006, we were flying to Red Bay, Ontario, for a wedding and had a layover in Winnipeg. In the time after our wedding and before giving birth to our son, I had been in contact with Catherine, and we were still trying to get in touch with Stella. For the first time in my life, I was on the other side of bipolar disorder, this time as a caregiver trying to lend support to a loved one (Catherine) as well as reach a dear friend in need of care (Stella). Catherine, who was still living in Winnipeg, met us at the airport during our layover. By then, our son, Noah, was only 2.5 months old, and given that I was nursing, my sleep was definitely suboptimal. By the time we arrived at the wedding destination, all the stress I had been under in the months prior felt compounded by the stress of the journey and travelling with a newborn. I became extremely irritable, didn't sleep well that night, and was increasingly anxious about being a bridesmaid in my friend's wedding the next day.

By mid-morning on the day of the wedding, it was clear that I was going manic. I was on my second night of little to no sleep; I was easily agitated; I was excited to see my friend and her fiancé and their family; I was excited to meet new people and be reunited with friends from naturopathic school; and I was anxious about my bridesmaid role. I had a heightened awareness. It was difficult for me to relax. As the day went on and we prepared for the wedding, I escalated into psychosis and began experiencing delusions at the hair salon. It became clear that I could not be in the wedding.

This would be the first episode I had ever had without being on any pharmaceutical medication. While it is unfortunate that this happened while I was at a friend's wedding, the upside was that there were many naturopathic doctors there to help me, including my husband. One in particular, Dr. Jason Hughes, was exceptional with his skills in grounding me and preventing me from following my psychotic thoughts too far down the rabbit hole. But the one thing that I kept repeating in the midst of my madness was that Stella was in the room. I kept repeating that she was there—and Dr. Hughes and Michael kept reassuring me that she wasn't. Eventually, they were able to calm me down enough (using my emergency stash of lorazepam and mega doses of melatonin) to avoid the need for me to go to the hospital.

The next day, we travelled to Toronto. When we got to our hotel, there was an urgent message from Catherine. When we reached her, she told us the news: Stella had committed suicide the night before. I literally dropped the phone and fell to the ground. A deep primal wail of pain welled out of me. I sobbed intensely. The aching pain that coursed through my heart and body upon hearing of Stella's tragic death was almost unbearable and like nothing I had ever experienced before. The previous night, I had constantly repeated that Stella was in the room and that she needed our help. I definitely feel like her soul was present where we were, or that I may have channelled her. I didn't understand why I had been so focused on her during my manic episode; perhaps it was just a coincidence. All I know is an amazing person was lost to suicide. She was a daughter, friend, clinician, and colleague who was dearly loved. She left a permanent imprint on our hearts. We will never forget her.

My only regret is that we didn't try harder to reach her and help her before she lost herself in the madness of her mind. In the end, Stella was seeing a psychiatrist, who had diagnosed her with anxiety and bipolar disorder type 2. Similar to hiding her lesbianism for so many years, according to Catherine, Stella had also been hiding that she was bipolar. She had said that she didn't want anyone to know this about her because she felt like no one would trust her as a practitioner. I can attest to the same fears. It is the fear of stigma and shame that steals the lives of many with mental illness. In Stella's case, the bigger problem was that this stigma prevented her from seeking out and accepting help soon enough. This fear was so tenacious in her that it blocked her from accepting help from Catherine or myself—both medical professionals who would have accepted her "label" or diagnosis.

2008

My last manic episode was in 2008. The common theme for each of the episodes from 2000 onward had been stress: financial stress, the stress of starting a new career when everyone else was excelling in theirs, the stress of comparing myself with others, the stress of getting married, of moving to a new city with no family support, of starting a family without the security of a full-time job, of starting a business—all of these undertakings were extremely taxing on my nervous system.

As recounted above, in the year after graduating from naturopathic medical school, I had moved twice, started a new career, married, become pregnant, written board exams, suffered extreme financial stress, given birth, gone on maternity leave, endured a manic episode, and lost a dear friend to suicide. I was off the stress scale! By the time 2008 came around, I was still feeling the financial pressures of starting a new business, and was still breastfeeding my 23-month old son and not getting enough sleep.

In April, Michael and Noah travelled with me to Vancouver so I could attend a naturopathic conference. Often when I travelled home, I had the tendency to overschedule myself, trying to visit with as many people (friends and family) as possible. In the week leading up to the trip, I hadn't been sleeping very well, and it only got worse once I arrived in Vancouver.

At that time in my life, it was hard for me to let go of an event after it happened. For example, if I went out for dinner with a group of friends, I would lie awake processing the evening, thinking about who said what and why they may have said what they did. Meditation, practising the Four Agreements (see below), and journalling are tools that have helped me tremendously in recent years; but in 2008, I only had journalling in my repertoire of stress management tools, and sometimes it just wasn't enough.

THE FOUR AGREEMENTS BY DON MIGUEL RUIZ

Be Impeccable with Your Word

Speak with integrity. Say only what you mean. Avoid using the word to speak against yourself or to gossip about others. Use the power of your word in the direction of truth and love.

Don't Take Anything Personally

Nothing others do is because of you. What others say and do is a projection of their own reality, their own dreams. When you are immune to the opinions and actions of others, you won't be the victim of needless suffering.

Don't Make Assumptions

Find the courage to ask questions and to express what you really want. Communicate with others as clearly as you can to avoid misunderstandings, sadness and drama. With just this one agreement, you can completely transform your life.

Always Do Your Best

Your best is going to change from moment to moment; it will be different when you are healthy as opposed to sick. Under any circumstance, simply do your best, and you will avoid self-judgment, self-abuse and regret.

SOURCE: The Four Agreements © 1997, Miguel Angel Ruiz, M.D. Reprinted by permission of Amber-Allen Publishing, Inc. San Rafael, CA www.amberallen.com. All rights reserved.

After a night of suboptimal sleep, I took to the Internet and sent an email to my family and in-laws about how I was truly feeling about my life and them. Raw honesty combined with a dose of hypomania is not always received so well, let me tell you. I attended the conference the next day, but became increasingly agitated and irritated as the day went on. I came across as irritable, confrontational and demanding. Since I wasn't wearing a name tag, the conference organizers didn't know my background, and given the circumstances, I was asked to leave. At this request, I created a huge disruption, became very vocal and did not go quietly. That night, we were supposed to meet my dad for dinner. When we got to the restaurant, the hostess said my dad had cancelled the reservation. I was furious. His actions and lack of communication struck my abandonment fears to the core. We left the restaurant and I dropped Michael and Noah off at Cheryl's house. I then raced in the rental car over to my dad's house in West Vancouver, escalating into mania as I drove. I am lucky I made it there alive.

When I got to my dad's house, I was in a state of distraught psychosis, imagining that he had cancelled the reservation because either he or my stepmother was sick. My dad would not let me in the house, and was yelling at me from behind the front door. He told me he had called the police. My heart sank at this news, given my previous experience with the police. He had also called Michael. I tried to remain as calm as possible while being locked out despite being in psychosis. This was also painfully difficult, not only because I was losing my mind, but because of the wide range and intensity of emotions I felt coursing through my veins: rage, frustration, abandonment, irritation, worry.

The police and Michael and Cheryl arrived within minutes of each other. I refused to look at or speak to the police. I pretended they weren't there and projected all my previous negative experiences onto them. I didn't want anything to do with them. Since the police were from West Vancouver, but the hospital I would need to go to was in downtown Vancouver (outside their jurisdiction), it was agreed that Michael and Cheryl would take me to emergency.

At one point in the admitting process, the nurse left me alone in the room. With my hospital bracelet on, I proceeded to walk out the front door of the hospital. I thought Michael and Cheryl had left me, and I did not want to be admitted and shot up with haloperidol (a powerful anti-psychotic). When the nurse discovered I wasn't there, she asked Michael and Cheryl, who were in the waiting room, where I was. They both stared at her in shock, saying that they thought I was with her. "Escape St. Paul's Hospital" swung into full operation. By this time, it was approaching 10 p.m., and it was a 10-kilometre walk to Cheryl's house, including a major bridge crossing. I didn't have any money for a cab. I decided to walk to another friend's house, since she lived a little closer. But to get to her house, I had to walk through Vancouver's Downtown Eastside.

If you have ever been to Vancouver, then you might know that the Downtown Eastside area is notorious for its open-air drug trade, sex work, and high rates of poverty, mental illness, infectious disease, and crime. In 1997, an epidemic of HIV infection and drug overdoses in the Downtown Eastside led to the declaration of a public health emergency. In recent years, the spread of infectious diseases has dramatically slowed, but the impacts of mental illness have reached a level that the city and police describe as a crisis, and overdoses of fentanyl have risen dramatically. At the time of writing this book, there is a fentanyl drug crisis happening in this area of Vancouver, as well as in other parts of Canada.

The Downtown Eastside is "home" to half of Vancouver's homeless. Many locals are nervous, frightened even, to walk through this part of town. But I have always looked at people as just that: people. And deep down, one of my fears was that I, too, would end up living on the streets in this part of town, given my mental illness. Some who are there have the same mental health issues that I have.

My walk to my friend's house was interesting, to say the least, especially in my state of psychosis. I talked to many homeless, mentally ill or addicted souls along the way. I was constantly asked for money or drugs, but since I genuinely didn't have either, I was left alone. I managed to make it safely to my destination just after midnight. Luckily, my friend was home, and still awake. She was surprised to see me. Interestingly enough, her mother also had bipolar disorder, so she knew how to handle me. She immediately turned off all stimulation—lights and TV—and spoke to me in an extremely gentle and calm tone of voice.

Meanwhile, after I had left the hospital, Michael and Cheryl had become frantic to find me. They were close to reporting me as a missing person. They had left the hospital and gone back to Cheryl's house in hopes they would find me there. After calming down at my friend's house, I asked her to drive me across town to Cheryl's. When I arrived, it was clear to me that I needed medical attention; I agreed to return to the hospital. Despite agreeing to receive emergency psychiatric medical care, I escalated into a rage, like I did in my very first episode. Similar to that episode, I was locked in a rubber room and separated from my loved ones. And just like before, when I had flushed my promise ring down the toilet, this time I flushed my wedding ring, as I was mad and upset with Michael for leaving me there. It was like a part of me forgot that I had agreed to be there. I felt abandoned again.

Upon getting discharged from the hospital, I learned that there had been complaints about my behaviour voiced by exhibitors at the conference, and some had suggested my licence be revoked.

As my friend Janet had explained when she came to help me during the 2003 manic episode at St. Paul's Hospital, it is a deeply profound experience to witness someone in mania. I recall that at the conference, I was easily triggered by aggressive energy, which led to my confrontational and disruptive behavior and my rather conspicuous removal from the venue.

It is difficult for the general public to differentiate between someone being belligerent and someone in genuine mental emotional distress due to mental illness. While I may have been viewed as a "bad apple" who was not fit to see patients or represent the naturopathic profession, this judgment was simply that: a judgment. Although I was dismayed by the exhibitors' reactions, which felt like a slap in the face, I can see their point of view. Given their complaints, I had to ask for letters of support from my psychiatrist and several colleagues in order to continue practising as a naturopathic doctor. This was more stress that I didn't need, and further highlights the ignorance of many people, including those working in the health care industry, with regards to mental illness.

That was my last manic episode to date.

(8)

If Money Didn't Matter

"In order to heal it, you need to reveal it. Healing happens when you return to yourself and let go of what no longer serves you."
DR. CHRIS

THAT BRINGS US to today. At the time of writing, I have been "stable" since 2008. Am I cured? Are we ever? The question of whether I am "healed" or "cured" from bipolar disorder is one that I wrestle with in my mind. Does the propensity to become unwell remain in the recesses of my mind? With the right combination of stress, will I go manic again?

Since being diagnosed with bipolar disorder type 1, I have lived in fear of mania. Much of the personal growth work I have done centres around acceptance, love and compassion for all aspects of my being—even those parts of myself that I have been afraid of, like mania. For now, I choose to believe that this part of me is managed through ensuring a proper diet, adequate sleep and stress management, which includes yoga, meditation, exercise, journalling, prayer and counselling.

The common theme running through all my manic episodes to date has been stress, and my quest to find answers for why mania occurs has led me to the adrenochrome and adrenolutin hypothesis of schizophrenia, which was first put forward by Dr. Hoffer in 1952.

71

The adrenochrome hypothesis

Essentially, adrenochrome is an intermediary by-product of the breakdown of adrenalin in the body. Dr. Hoffer hypothesized that some individuals are unable to clear adrenalin from their systems quickly enough, and it becomes oxidized, forming a free radical. It is as if adrenochrome builds up to a toxic level and floods the brain, where it saturates receptors and has a drug-like effect, triggering psychosis. Using a car analogy, if you flood your car engine with gas, it won't run. This is what happens in the mind when it is flooded by adrenochrome: it can't run properly either.

Dr. Hoffer concluded: "The adrenochrome hypothesis accounts for the syndrome of schizophrenia more accurately than do any of the competing hypotheses. Unfortunately, the many leads developed by the adrenochrome hypothesis have been neglected by research institutions for a number of reasons. The critical and hostile attitude of the professional associations and granting agencies discouraged scientists from entering this difficult but challenging field."

However, the fact that the adrenochrome hypothesis has not been properly researched does not mean it is incorrect. Time will tell. It is a good, testable hypothesis, and further research should be directed toward this theory. Why, then, has it been ignored for nearly 30 years?

In his writing, Dr. Hoffer suggested that despite gaining a certain amount of notoriety in the beginning, the adrenochrome hypothesis was quickly shot down by American psychiatrists at the National Institute of Mental Health. He concluded: "A medical historian may one day be able to examine the issues more capably. In our opinion, there were two main classes of opinion: scientific and political. The political opposition prevented any serious examination of the consequences of the adrenochrome hypothesis. No ideas spring forth from a vacuum. All new ideas must confront the establishment of ideas until a new paradigm is created. But the establishment of ideas may be so pervasive and powerful it is able to swamp and overwhelm new ideas. The adrenochrome hypothesis of schizophrenia attacked, head-on, several establishments."

In my own case, and those of my patients who experience psychosis, this hypothesis seems plausible. I think it is important for people to understand that medicine doesn't really know why mental illness happens. Scientists don't fully understand how the brain works. This was highlighted to me in an interview that I saw on CBC TV's *The National* after Robin Williams committed suicide. The psychiatrist interviewed for the segment said: "We don't know why this happens or how the brain works." I found that comment disheartening, to say the least. I put up my hands in despair and said, "What are you guys doing then? Here we are prescribing all these medications and we don't really know how the brain works!"

I've also heard Dr. Daniel Amen say at a lecture that psychiatrists are the only medical specialists who don't look at the organ they are treating—cardiologists look at images of the heart and nephrologists look at images of the kidneys (and so on), but psychiatrists don't actually look at the brain.

My journey—and your plan

My journey to regain my mental health has resulted in this plan that I am sharing so that you, in turn, can regain yours. The next chapters will explain how to support your body's three macrosystems—neurotransmitters, the neuroendocrine system, and the organs of detoxification—so that you can support your mood. I suggest supporting them by addressing the foundations of health:

- Diet
- Sleep
- Exercise
- Managing stress

And by addressing your:

- Thoughts
- Emotions
- Behaviours and reactions
- Environment
- Spirituality
- Love and compassion for yourself

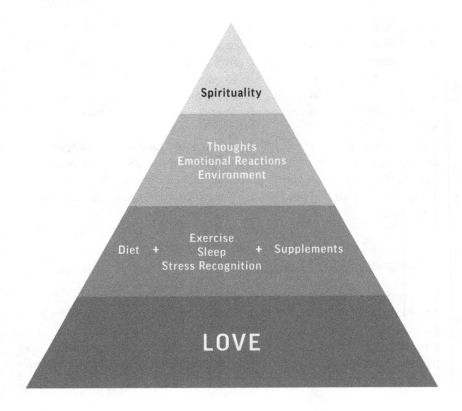

When working with patients, my ultimate goal is to teach them to love and accept themselves. I believe that, at the end of the day, it all comes down to that.

O▬ *In your **Moving Beyond** journal, write about which of the 10 areas are working well in your life. Are there any that need improvement?*

I also explain to patients that the goal is to get people to achieve optimal functioning, or 10 out of 10 health.

Many patients want to get to 10 out of 10 health immediately. Most expect the road to recovery to be a straight line from points A to Z that happens in a time frame of yesterday. We all know this is not realistic, but it is truly how many people feel and what they expect. In reality, the road to recovery is not a straight line as outlined in the diagram, but there is some back and forth, and it can look more like this:

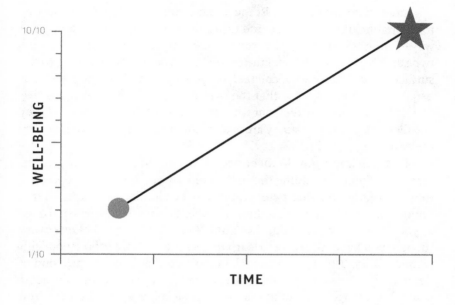

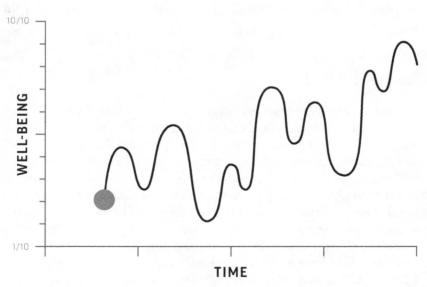

Understand that just as Rome wasn't built in a day, your journey to mental health may take some time. There may be bumps along the way—it might be four steps forward, one step back, two steps forward, two steps back—as you "peel the onion" and your emotions come to the surface to heal. At times, it can feel like you aren't making progress—but usually, it will be the case that the overall trajectory has been positive. People know how they feel, but what they don't realize is how good they can feel. They may think they are at a 10 out of 10 in health, but in reality, they are at a 5 out of 10.

I find it is important to meet people where they are on the road to recovery. If you are reading this and would say you are 10/10 depressed, then your judgment and perceptions may be clouded or distorted. It is important to understand that this is not *you*. This is what depression does *to* you. You *can* change your thoughts. You don't have to believe every thought you have. You have to learn to become objective about your subjective reality. When you are stuck in it, it is difficult to see the cloud of depression in front of your eyes; it's so thick that you become the cloud. It is important to understand that on a soul level, *you* are still there. You are behind the cloud. And that cloud will lift and the sun will appear again in your life.

Taking the first step

The first step on a new path is always the hardest to take. Make it a small one, and you will be surprised that, in time, you will be running down the road of recovery. Remember that there may be potholes and it may feel like the journey is long and slow at times. Trust in the healing process, be patient, and you will get "there." There is no quick-fix solution to multifactorial conditions. Everyone needs to find his or her own balance point in life. Don't compare yourself with others. Trust in your own intuitive self and the inherent healing powers you have at your fingertips while working with experienced health care professionals.

Most people have addictions, issues, and things to get over, learn or adjust to. Life is about how we navigate the waves of our lives. It really is about the journey, not the destination. For most of my life, I lived for the destination while ignoring the journey. Now, I am learning to enjoy the journey as much as I appreciate the destination. I was recently asked to explain in a few words what I do. My response was: "I help people make peace with the present moment—piece by piece."

So far, you have read about my mental health challenges, and how I was on and off antidepressant, anti-anxiolytic and mood stabilizing medications for 15 years. Every time I went off them, I ended up depressed and anxious, and every time I was prescribed them, things would get moderately better. But the fact that I would get unwell again upon stopping them forced me to realize that I wasn't dealing with the root cause; I was just masking the symptoms. You have probably heard a similar analogy involving a car: when the engine isn't working properly, a light will come on, but if you ignore the light by cutting the wire (which is analogous to taking medication), pretty soon the car may stop running altogether because you never looked under the hood for the source of the problem.

To give another analogy: if you continually throw garbage outside your kitchen window, there will eventually be flies to contend with. You can deal with the flies by spraying poison on them, and even spray the garbage pile itself. This is like using antibiotics or antidepressants. Or, you can clean up the garbage and stop throwing more on the pile. Not only will the flies go away, but the kitchen will smell better. This is the naturopathic approach: clean up the garbage. If you do, the flies won't come back when the poisons wear off. Nor will they build up a resistance to the poisons.

The first step to regaining your mental health is to recognize that the physical building blocks for forming neurotransmitters come from foods and nutraceuticals. Most people come to me because they want an alternative to pharmaceuticals. Some of my patients have been on medication for more than 20 years. Others may not be on any medication, but feel anxious or depressed and want to know if there is something they can do to avoid starting an antidepressant or anti-anxiolytic.

No matter how you are feeling, I know that if you follow the steps outlined in the subsequent chapters, you will feel better than you do today.

(9)

The Big Picture:
Macrosystems Overview

"Play with the idea that your life has infinite possibilities."
DR. CHRIS

THUS FAR, I'VE told you a lot about me—about my struggles with my mental health and all the labels I've been assigned. Now I want to explain how you can overcome your own labels, and move beyond them to a place of balance and peace. Ultimately, what I will teach you is how to make peace with the present moment. All you have to do is implement the suggestions in the following chapters. I hope you are as excited as I am about the possibilities for your life!

First, it is important to recognize that we have physical, mental, emotional and spiritual aspects to ourselves.

Western medicine places a great deal of emphasis on the physical—and it is important to understand that if that is all we focus on, we miss most of what makes all of us human. It is my goal to address all aspects with patients. In Western medicine, the underlying assumption is that if we prescribe the right pharmaceutical, nutraceutical or botanical remedy, we can correct the imbalance and the person will feel better. In many cases, this is all that is required. However, in other instances, it is necessary to address all aspects. By correcting underlying physical imbalances first, you will be in a better place to address the mental, emotional and

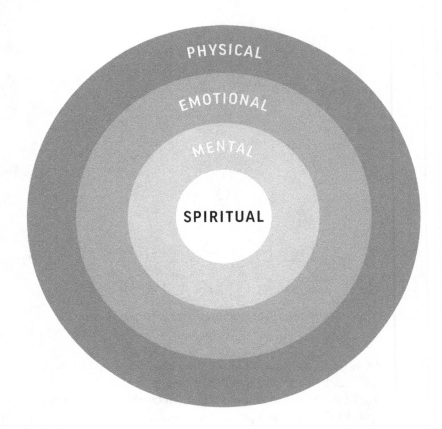

spiritual aspects of health. I also feel that if all we look at is the physical level, we may never address the root cause of mental dis-ease, which can originate in one of the other areas. By taking a naturopathic approach to mental health and addressing all aspects of a person, not just one part of the puzzle (when you only look at the physical level) but a truly holistic approach is achieved.

The physical level

What is important to understand about the physical level, especially since our Western medical system is primarily focused on this area, is that you are made up of three macrosystems: 1) neurotransmitters;

2) your neuroendocrine system; and 3) your organs of detoxification. All of the chemical messengers made by our macrosystems interact with each other. Part of the problem with our current medical system is that we have created specialties for various health conditions. For example, if you are depressed, you see a psychiatrist; if you have hormone problems, you see an endocrinologist; if you have a heart problem, you see a cardiologist. We have compartmentalized our health into silos, and no one is looking at you as an entire system. This is important to understand, as everything in your body is interacting. While your neurotransmitters may originate in your brain, they can cause you to have digestive concerns, which will affect how your liver and hormones function, which can lead you to have heart problems. In naturopathic medicine, we do not defer your care to a different department because we view you as one entity.

When dealing with mental health, it is important to take a thorough case history in order to investigate which macrosystems are playing a role. Bear in mind that there is often more than one thing going on in the body at a time. In practice, I find that all three macrosystems may need to be addressed. As such, for optimal mental health, it is important to determine which neurotransmitters and neurohormones are out of balance. Typically, in psychiatry, medications are used to restore balance to neurotransmitters. There are six neurotransmitters: two that are inhibitory (serotonin and gamma amino butyric acid [GABA]) and four that are excitatory (norepinephrine, acetylcholine, dopamine and glutamate).

The neurotransmitter most commonly implicated when someone has both depression and anxiety is serotonin. This is why there is an entire medication class dedicated to supporting serotonin called selective serotonin reuptake inhibitors (SSRIs). These include medications such as citalopram (Celexa), escitalopram (Cipralex), fluoxetine (Prozac), fluvoxamine (Luvox), paroxetine (Paxil), vortioxetine (Trintellix) and sertraline (Zoloft).

What is also important to investigate is whether the neuroendocrine system—which consists of the hypothalamus, pituitary, thyroid, adrenals and ovaries (in women) or testes (in men)—is contributing to one's mood.* Each of these glands produces hormones, and imbalances in them can

---

* Some also include the pancreas and heart in the neuroendocrine system, as these organs also produce chemical messengers that can have an effect on mood and appetite.

result in the symptoms of depression and/or anxiety. What happened for me when I started Dr. Hoffer's protocol was that instead of having a mood disturbance for the entire month, I noticed a considerable improvement in my mood for half of the month. For the two weeks prior to my menstrual cycle, I would still experience mood swings. This was a clue that my hormones were playing a role in my mental health.

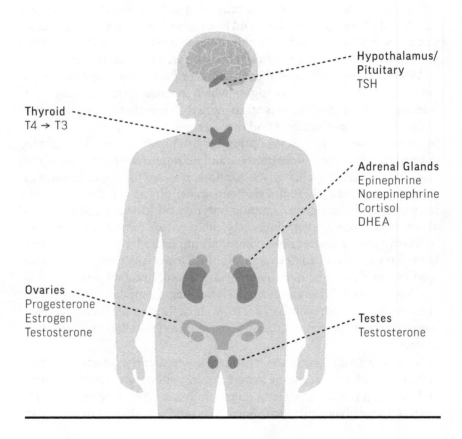

Hypothalamus/
Pituitary
TSH

Thyroid
T4 → T3

Adrenal Glands
Epinephrine
Norepinephrine
Cortisol
DHEA

Ovaries
Progesterone
Estrogen
Testosterone

Testes
Testosterone

Essentially, all the neurotransmitters and the neurohormones are like a symphony operating in unison to orchestrate your life. The following tables outline symptoms that are possible if you have hormone imbalances.

NEUROTRANSMITTER	CONDITIONS IN WHICH IT IS INVOLVED
Serotonin contributes to various functions, such as regulating body temperature, sleep, mood, appetite and pain.	Depression, suicide, anxiety, impulsive behaviour and aggression all appear to involve imbalances in serotonin.
GABA is an inhibitory neurotransmitter that is very widely distributed in the neurons of the cortex. GABA contributes to motor control, vision and many other cortical functions. It also regulates anxiety.	Some drugs that increase the level of GABA in the brain are used to treat epilepsy and calm trembling in people suffering from Huntington's disease. It is also used to treat anxiety.
Glutamate is a major excitatory neurotransmitter associated with learning and memory.	It is also thought to be associated with Alzheimer's disease, whose first symptoms include memory malfunctions.
Norepinephrine is important for attentiveness, emotions, sleeping, dreaming and learning. It is also released as a hormone into the bloodstream, where it causes blood vessels to contract and heart rate to increase.	Norepinephrine plays a role in mood disorders, such as bipolar disorder.

NEUROTRANSMITTER	CONDITIONS IN WHICH IT IS INVOLVED
Dopamine helps control movement and posture. It also modulates mood and plays a central role in positive reinforcement and dependency.	The loss of dopamine in certain parts of the brain causes the muscle rigidity typical of Parkinson's disease. There is a connection with dopamine and addiction, as well as schizophrenia.
Acetylcholine triggers muscle contraction and stimulates the excretion of certain hormones. In the central nervous system, it is involved in wakefulness, attentiveness, anger, aggression, sexuality and thirst, among other things.	Alzheimer's disease is associated with a lack of acetylcholine in certain regions of the brain.

ESTROGEN

Deficiency	Excess
Hot flashes	Mood swings/irritability
Night sweats	Fibrocystic and/or tender breasts
Vaginal dryness	Water retention
Memory lapses/foggy thinking	Foggy thinking
Incontinence	**Anxiety**
Tearfulness	Weight gain (hips)
Depression	Menstrual bleeding changes
Disturbed sleep	Headaches
Heart palpitations	Uterine fibroids
Bone loss	Cold body temperature
	Fatigue/insomnia

PROGESTERONE

Deficiency	Excess
Mood swings/irritability	Drowsiness
Fibrocystic and/or tender breasts	Breast swelling
Water retention	Nausea
Foggy thinking	**Depression**
Anxiety	Foggy thinking
Weight gain (hips)	Oily skin
Menstrual bleeding changes	Increased acne
Headaches	Excess facial hair
Uterine fibroids	
Cold body temperature	
Fatigue/insomnia	

CORTISOL

Deficiency	Excess
Fatigue	**Irritable**
Allergies	Feeling "tired but wired"
Aching muscles	or "burnt out"
Feeling cold	Weight gain (waist)
Neck stiffness	Loss of muscle mass
Increased infections	Bone loss
Morning sluggishness	High blood pressure
Feeling "burned out"	Insulin resistance
Low sex drive	Low sex drive
Feeling unable to cope	Impaired memory
Depression/anxiety	Loss of scalp hair

DHEA*

Deficiency	Excess
Depression/anxiety	Greasy hair and skin
Frequent illness	Acne
Joint pain	Excess body odour
Decreased muscle mass	Increased ratio of testosterone:
Decreased bone density	estrogen
Fatigue	
Decreased libido (women)	*In women*: increased facial and
Increased risk of breast cancer,	abdominal hair, a deeper voice,
cardiovascular disease and	male-pattern baldness, muscu-
osteoporosis	larity, Adam's apple enlargement,
Hair loss (scalp, armpits & pubic)	decreased breast size
Cellulitis	
Decreased noise resistance	
Dry skin and dry eyes	

---

* DHEA is short for dehydroepiandrosterone. It is an anti-aging hormone.

TESTOSTERONE

Deficiency	Excess
Fatigue	Acne
Depression	Oily skin
Decreased sex drive	Excess facial/body hair
Sleep disturbances	Weight gain
Decreased muscle mass	Insulin resistance
Muscle aches/stiffness	Polycystic ovaries
Memory lapses/foggy thinking/ poor concentration	**Irritability**
Bone loss	Loss of scalp hair

In men: Erectile dysfunction &/ or problems urinating, weight gain &/or breast enlargement

In women: Vaginal dryness/ incontinence

THYROID HORMONES

Deficiency *(Hypothyroid)*	Excess *(Hyperthyroid)*
Fatigue/exhaustion	**Mood swings**
Anxiety & panic attacks	**Irritability**
Heat or cold intolerance	**Nervousness**
Hair loss	Hand tremors
Dry skin & hair	Dry skin
Easy weight gain	**Weight loss**
Insomnia	**Trouble sleeping**
Constipation	Increased bowel movements
Flushing	Rapid heartbeat
Allergies	Muscle weakness
Acne	Dizziness
Headaches	Itching & hives
Slow healing	Shortness of breath
Brain fog (decreased memory)	Problems with fertility
Depression	Possible increase in blood sugar
Dry eyes/blurred vision	Vision changes
Low motivation & ambition	Light or missed periods

Understanding macrosystems

As mentioned, there are three macrosystems to address: 1) neurotransmitters; 2) the neuroendocrine or hormonal system; and 3) organs of detoxification. The third macrosystem, the organs of detoxification, plays an important role in our general health and well-being. The organs of detoxification consist of the following: liver, kidneys, colon, lungs, skin and lymphatic system. While they are all important, the key ones that I will address are the liver and colon. If these are not working properly, you can have the following symptoms:

- Abdominal bloating
- Constipation
- Excess abdominal fat
- Acid reflux/heartburn
- Acne/rosacea/eczema or itchy, blotchy skin
- Unexplained weight gain or inability to lose weight even with caloric restriction
- Fatigue
- High cholesterol and triglycerides
- Mood swings and depression
- Hormone imbalances

For many people, the reality is that all three of the macrosystems need to be addressed. This is because there are many probable causes for mental health conditions.

Mental health conditions: Possible causal factors

- Deficiencies in vitamin B6, folic acid, vitamin B12, vitamin B1, iron, zinc, magnesium, vitamin D and/or vitamin C
- Excessive consumption of methylxanthines, which are found in such foods as coffee, black tea, pop (cola) and chocolate
- Excessive consumption of simple sugars (this can trigger hypoglycemic reactions—i.e., low blood sugar—and result in mood imbalances, such as depression, anxiety and bipolar disorder)
- Imbalances in brain neurotransmitters
- Certain drugs, including oral contraceptives, alcohol, nicotine, cannabis, caffeine, corticosteroids, beta blockers, and other anti-

hypertensive medications (oral contraceptives may lead to depression in a significant number of women because they create deficiencies in vitamin B6, folic acid, vitamin B1, vitamin C, and vitamin B12; they may also cause serotonin levels to drop)

- Hormone imbalances (i.e., hypothyroidism), food allergies or sensitivities, and heavy metals

The question of genetics often comes up in discussions of predisposition to mental health conditions.* Many individuals who suffer from recurrent episodes of depression have a parent who has also experienced depression. While this is a common explanation given to patients, I feel the gene theory leaves people feeling like they are victims, as if they are helpless and unable to change. Personally, I do not believe we are at the mercy of our genes. I subscribe to the theory that "genes load the gun; lifestyle pulls the trigger." This is based on the work of Bruce Lipton in *The Biology of Belief* and the field of epigenetics. Epigenetics is the study of how factors in the environment can switch genes on or off.

WHAT IS EPIGENETICS?

Epigenetics is the study of biological mechanisms that will affect gene expression (active versus inactive genes) that does not involve changes to the underlying DNA sequence. This in turn affects how cells read the genes and subsequently how they produce proteins. Epigenetic change is a regular and natural occurrence, but it can also be influenced by several factors, including age, the environment/lifestyle and disease state. Here are a few important points about epigenetics:

- **Epigenetics controls genes.** Certain circumstances in life can cause genes to be turned off (becoming dormant) or turned on (becoming active).

- **Epigenetics is everywhere.** What you eat, where you live, who you interact with, when you sleep, how you exercise, even aging—all of these can

---

* I know there is much research about methylation pathways and genetic single nucleotide polymorphisms that might be the cause of mental illness, and I am not discrediting the work of science in this area. There is also the immune/inflammation theory of mental illness, which is also plausible.

eventually cause chemical modifications around the genes that will turn those genes on or off over time.

- **Epigenetics makes us unique.** The different combinations of genes that are turned on or off is what makes each one of us unique. Research is now showing that some epigenetic changes can be inherited.

Lab tests can be helpful in assessing the function of the macrosystems. There are three ways to test hormone levels: blood, urine and saliva.

When working with patients, I typically start with current blood work to assess levels of certain nutrients (i.e., vitamin B12 and iron), hormones, cholesterol levels, liver enzymes and thyroid function. One of the differences between NDs and MDs is our approach to interpreting blood test results. Usually, MDs wait until you are outside a reference range to make recommendations. NDs practise functional, or optimal, medicine, which means we don't wait until you are outside a reference range to make suggestions. Instead, we look at where you are in a reference range and make recommendations accordingly. By doing so, we can help prevent deficiencies and promote optimal health. Naturopathic doctors also offer food intolerance testing, essential and toxic mineral testing, comprehensive digestive stool analysis, neurotransmitter testing, and organic acid testing.

My philosophy is to start with an overview of how the macrosystems are functioning as determined by a thorough patient case history and assessment of blood work. Additional testing may be needed, but I don't believe in looking for a needle in a haystack. I don't support a reductionist approach, which involves elaborate biochemical tests. This often leads to over-diagnosis and over-treatment. I am not averse to testing, but my concern lies in the way testing is contextualized, as I don't believe the roots of a person's emotional suffering will necessarily be found through testing.

The good news is that the probable causes of mental health are treatable. Once you start supporting the macrosystems, you will feel better! The way I go about supporting these three macrosystems is by addressing the fundamentals of health:

1. Diet
2. Sleep
3. Exercise
4. Stress
5. Thoughts
6. Emotions
7. Behaviours and reactions
8. Environment
9. Spirituality
10. Love and compassion for yourself.

(10)

Diet—You Are
What You Eat, Part 1

*"Eating fast food might save you time and money in the short
run, but it will cost you your life in the long run."*

DR. CHRIS

YOUR TISSUES, ORGANS, bones, blood, brain and every cell that
makes up those parts of you are created from what you put in your
body. You have probably heard the expressions "You are what you
what you eat," "The car won't run if you don't put the right fuel in the
tank," or "Garbage in/garbage out." Well, this is absolutely true when
it comes to your health and nutrition. I am not convinced that you are
anxious and depressed because you have a deficiency of Prozac. You are
anxious and depressed, perhaps, because your body is not supporting the
pathway to make serotonin on its own, because:

- You do not have the essential nutrients to do so, or
- You are missing the nutritional cofactors along the pathway to sero-
  tonin, or
- You are deficient in vitamin B3, or
- You are stressed out and forming quinolinic acid instead.

There are also a number of other factors that can decrease the amount
of serotonin in your body. They include:

- Seasonal affective disorder
- An excess of estrogen
- A low-protein or low-carbohydrate diet
- Chronic stress
- Excessive caffeine or alcohol consumption
- Thyroid disease
- Habitual use of tranquilizers, benzodiazepines or sleeping pills
- Menopause
- A deficiency of beneficial gut flora, which impacts the gut-brain axis

Or perhaps you don't have a serotonin manufacturing problem at all, but due to heavy metals and endocrine disruptors in the environment, there are other molecules blocking receptors so that serotonin can't get inside the cell to do its job. In that case, it isn't actually a deficiency problem, but a binding problem. Alternatively, another neurotransmitter or neurohormone could be deficient, especially when a specific class of medications has been tried with no success, such as selective serotonin reuptake inhibitors (SSRIs).

Understanding serotonin deficiency

In psychiatry, depression and anxiety are often viewed as deficiency problems. The belief is you aren't making enough of the neurotransmitter (typically serotonin) and that is why you need medication. It is important to understand the biochemical pathways in the body and what nutritional precursors are necessary to form these molecules.

Serotonin deficiency is most often assumed to be the culprit when it comes to depression, anxiety, bipolar disorder and eating disorders. This is the neurotransmitter pathway that I ensure is supported in patients when they present with either depression and/or depression along with anxiety or one of the other aforementioned mental health concerns. What is important to know is that serotonin is derived from tryptophan. When I ask patients if they have heard of tryptophan, many say, "Yes, is that in turkey?" And it is. Tryptophan is an *essential* amino acid, with the key word being "essential."

The *Merriam-Webster Dictionary* defines essential as: extremely important and necessary. What that means is we cannot make it on our own. We need to get tryptophan from our diet. In total, there are

20 amino acids required for human life, and of these, nine are essential amino acids. The nine essential amino acids, which we cannot make on our own, are histidine, isoleucine, leucine, lysine, methionine, phenylalanine, threonine, tryptophan and valine.

It is important to your recovery that you stop and fully fathom the magnitude of this. The key neurotransmitter that is needed to support your mood is derived from an essential amino acid that you can't make. You must get it from your diet. From a root cause perspective, taking medication may not be a permanent solution to your problems if you never fix the underlying biological terrain of your body to support the production of serotonin and other neurotransmitters. It is entirely possible that you are mentally unwell because you have an essential amino acid deficiency. It is important to understand that every morsel of food, every liquid and every substance that enters your body informs your body in one way or another. The key is to make sure that you are sending your body the right messages.

As you can see from the following diagram, there are three directions in which tryptophan can go when it enters the body. First, it will go to make niacin (vitamin B3). Niacin is used in every cell to make adenosine triphosphate (ATP), which is the energy currency cells use to stay alive. Making sure we have enough niacin to support the cellular functioning of

Serotonin Pathway

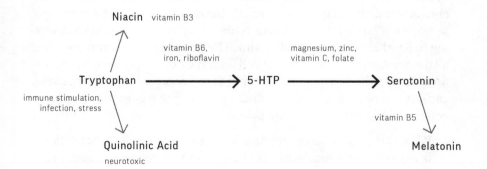

our organs is the body's priority. It is more important to keep our hearts beating and our lungs breathing than it is for us to feel good. Another important note about niacin is that it supports the elimination of glutamate, which is an excitatory neurotransmitter. Glutamate can affect our ability to utilize folate, which is also an essential nutrient required to maintain our mental health.

Once we have adequate niacin stores, we want tryptophan to go down the pathway to make 5-hydroxytryptophan (5-HTP), a precusor to making serotonin (the feel-good neurotransmitter) and ultimately melatonin (the sleep hormone). We also must ensure we have adequate amounts of the nutritional cofactors (vitamin B6, magnesium, vitamin C, zinc, etc.) so we can convert tryptophan to serotonin. However, if we are under a tremendous amount of stress, then tryptophan can be shunted to the kynurenic pathway in the body. Instead of being converted to serotonin, tryptophan is converted to quinolinic acid. Research demonstrates that increased quinolinic acid levels correlate with increased depressive symptoms. If there is reason to suspect this, an organic acid test can be helpful, as it will tell you if you have nutritional deficiencies as well as urinary metabolites of serotonin and quinolinic acid. Niacin is also important in this pathway, as it inhibits a gene that feeds in to the kynurenic pathway. This pathway ends up depleting tryptophan levels, which further decreases serotonin, contributing to depression and anxiety. Niacin slows the loss of tryptophan by directing it toward serotonin formation.

From a pharmaceutical perspective, SSRI medications serve to increase the length of time that serotonin is available in the synaptic cleft between two neurons in the brain. SSRI medications are based on the chemical imbalance theory of mental illness: that you don't have enough serotonin. The way it works in our brain is you have one neuron connecting to another neuron (see diagram). The transmitting neuron contains all the serotonin. Essentially, the cell fires, the doors open, and serotonin floats across the synaptic cleft to bind to the receptor on the other side, causing the next neuron to fire. And down the line it goes in the brain. A couple of points to take into consideration:

- What if it is not a serotonin deficiency problem at all? What if there is enough serotonin, but it can't bind to the receptor because there is something blocking it? There are many neurotoxins and heavy metals in the environment that do just that. So, you may not have a manufacturing problem at all, but rather a getting-in-the-door or binding problem.

- It is important to understand or ask yourself what serotonin is made from. How does the body make it? As discussed, it comes from tryptophan.

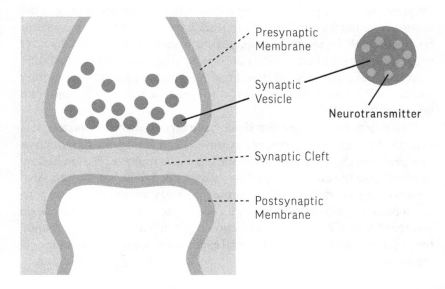

Presynaptic Membrane

Synaptic Vesicle

Neurotransmitter

Synaptic Cleft

Postsynaptic Membrane

Diet and serotonin

We have to remember that if mental health issues are due to a deficiency problem, diet has to be addressed to ensure that foods high in tryptophan, vitamin B6, magnesium, vitamin C, vitamin B3, iron, riboflavin, folate and zinc are being consumed in sufficient quantities. It is important to support serotonin from the beginning of its pathway versus its end point.

Another important consideration is the role of chemicals from the environment and the possibility that they can block receptors, preventing neurotransmitters from entering the cell. It is possible that you are making enough serotonin, but it can't get into the cell. From a root cause perspective, removing the chemicals that are blocking the receptors is the solution; simply providing the body with more serotonin will not solve the problem. This is important to consider if you are taking antidepressants and not feeling any better. See Chapter 16 for more information on the role of the environment.

As mentioned, in addition to serotonin, there are other neurotransmitters that play a role in mood, such as GABA (gamma amino butyric acid) and dopamine. If anxiety is the primary issue—and not depression—then I support the GABA pathway using nutraceuticals such as GABA, glycine, inositol, vitamin B6 and herbs. Often, addiction is involved as a concomitant factor with depression, anxiety, eating disorders and bipolar disorder, suggesting the neurotransmitter dopamine is involved. Since dopamine is an excitatory neurotransmitter, I find it is best to support the inhibitory pathways (i.e., serotonin and GABA) for the first few months and then reassess.

This is especially important if you have bipolar disorder, as overstimulation of the excitatory neurotransmitters can contribute to psychosis. The caveat to this may be if someone has had a major addiction history, in which case the dopamine pathway might need to be considered. Also, the cofactors needed for the dopamine pathway are similar to the serotonin pathway, which explains why I see improvement when I work on serotonin first. Ultimately, if addiction is playing a role in one's mental health, then counselling is an integral aspect to gaining mental emotional freedom.

How to eat

Although it's important to know what to eat to help these pathways run smoothly, first let's establish some guidelines on *how* to eat.

Step 1: Cook

Diet is the foundation of health! Remember, "You are what you eat." I'll add to that by saying that not only are you what you eat, but you are what you absorb and what you don't excrete. Many NDs feel that the root of all illness starts in the gut; heal the gut and you can heal anything.

Everything that passes through your mouth informs your body. In our modern society, we are often missing the first step in the digestive process: cooking. Digestion starts with the sense of smell, when we are preparing our food. This sends a signal to the brain that food is coming.

The brain sends a message to the stomach along the vagus nerve to get ready for the food to arrive. This first step is missing for most of us, as we no longer spend 20 to 60 minutes preparing our food. Instead, we unwrap something and down the hatch it goes. As a result, many of us have digestive complaints such as gas, bloating, heartburn, diarrhea or loose stool, constipation and nausea.

Ideally, I want you to cook at least one meal per day. There are two important branches to your autonomic nervous system: the sympathetic and parasympathetic branches. When we are stressed, we activate our sympathetic side, and when we are relaxed, we engage the parasympathetic branch. To work properly, certain functions in the body require you to be in a parasympathetic state. Digestion is a key function that requires a parasympathetic state. This means we need to be in a calm, relaxed state when we eat to get the maximum benefit from food. Many health experts focus on the quality of the food, but the emotional state you are in when you eat is equally important.

Step 2: Pause before you eat

Since digestion is a parasympathetic process, Step 2 is to take a few deep, rhythmic breaths before you eat to shift yourself into a relaxed state. This is especially important if you skipped Step 1 and didn't cook your food. Spend a few extra minutes thinking about all the steps involved before the food arrived on your plate: where it came from, who grew it and prepared it for you. Visualize your stomach being ready to receive the food before you even take one bite. Saying "grace" or enjoying a moment of appreciation before eating is a great way of pausing before consuming.

Step 3: Chew—and chew some more

When you do finally eat, there are a few key steps involved:

Put your fork down between bites.

Thoroughly chew your food: you want to make your solids liquid before swallowing. I encourage everyone to chew as many times as it takes to make your food liquid, whether that's 20, 40, 60, 80 or 100 times.

Don't talk with your mouth full. Focus on chewing and being present with your food.

If you are full, you don't need to finish all that is on your plate.

Step 4: Relax

The key to relaxing during mealtimes is to sit down when you eat and not do anything else, i.e., don't multitask. When you eat, just eat. Don't talk on the phone, watch TV, read or work. Remember, we need to be in a calm, relaxed state to aid digestion.

Mindful eating

The reason for these steps is to stop you from eating unconsciously. The idea is to be present and eat mindfully. When you do that, you are less likely to over-consume and more likely to get the maximum nutritional benefit from your food. You can have a pleasant conversation with someone while eating, as long as you remain calm.

The other important reason for these steps is that the more aware you are and the more time you take to eat, the greater the chances that you will recognize the "full" signal when it is activated.

There are many myths around eating, some of which might be guiding your beliefs around food, such as:

1. I need to eat everything I put on my plate.
2. I must eat because the clock tells me to.
3. I must avoid certain foods because they are bad for me.
4. It is hard to lose weight.
5. Cooking for one person is boring and not fun.
6. Nutrition is confusing; I don't know what to eat.

☛ *Take some time to write in your **Moving Beyond** journal about any beliefs that may be guiding your eating or your desire to lose weight.*

It is important to note that profitability drives our society and that it, not your nutritional health, is the key motivating force behind the food industry. In packaged food, food manufacturers manipulate three nutrients—sugar, fat and salt—so that we will become addicted to their products. Foods that contain high levels of sugar, fat and salt are intensely marketed; often, advertising influences our diet and health more than information from health professionals. As food technology has advanced, health life has been replaced by shelf life. Technological developments have provided benefits, but most often I find the mass processing of food is in the best interests of convenience and time, not nutrition or our mental well-being and mood.

What to eat—and how to know what you're eating

When it comes to food and eating right, I find many people are unclear about how to read food labels and what "types" of food to eat. Here is what I explain to my patients:

- There are three macromolecules: fat, protein and carbohydrates. All three are important to our well-being.
- Each macromolecule can be divided into two "micro-molecule" categories:
  - FAT = saturated "bad" fat and polyunsaturated "good" or "essential" fat
  - PROTEIN = non-essential and essential amino acids
  - CARBOHYDRATES = refined and complex carbohydrates

The idea is to eat more of the essential fats and proteins, as well as complex carbohydrates, and limit the "bad" foods. We need to do this because our body cannot make these essential molecules. That is why they are termed "essential," and we must get them from our diets or nature. The easiest way to do this is to shop only around the perimeter of the grocery store. If you must go up and down the aisles, choose boxed, canned or processed foods with fewer than five ingredients. When you are reading ingredients, start from the end of the list and read backwards. The first warning sign that a food isn't a good idea is a series of fancy words on the label that you have never heard of and can't pronounce. You want your food to fuel you and satisfy your hunger, not burden your organs of detoxification and fill up your fat cells.

The next challenge for most people is really a simple math equation. Food is measured in calories but listed on labels as calories per gram. So, for the three macronutrients, you need to remember two numbers: nine calories/gram for fats and four calories/gram for protein and carbohydrates. The problem with nutrition labels is that they list total calories as a percentage of daily value, but many of us have a different "daily value."

For example, my daily value for the three food groups is a balance of 30% complex carbohydrates, 30% protein (ensuring more essential proteins) and 30% essential polyunsaturated fat (primarily omega 3), with the last 10% of my daily calories coming from "fun" foods. Here is an example of how to make the calculations using a label from an energy bar:

Listed on Label	Conversion to Actual Calories Consumed	% of Nutrient in Food
Total calories: 243 calories per 55 g serving If the serving is 55 g, it follows:		
Fat 11 g - saturated fat 1.5 g - trans fat 0 g	11 g of fat × 9 calories/g = 99 calories from fat (Most of this fat is the "good" or essential fat. This is a good thing.)	99 calories/243 total calories = 40.7%
Carbohydrates 29 g - fibre 2 g - sugar 14 g	29 g of carbohydrates × 4 calories/g = 116 calories from carbohydrates	116 calories/243 total calories = 47.7%
Protein 7 g	7 g of protein × 4 calories/ g = 28 calories	28 calories/243 total calories = 11.6%
		Total Calories: **99 + 116 + 28 =** **243 = 100%**

The questions you need to ask yourself are: 1) Does this food choice fit into my overall eating objectives? 2) Will it help me reach my goal?

In the above example, even though the energy bar does not break down into the perfect 30-30-30 ratio, it meets my other food criteria: high in essential fats, high in complex carbohydrates, a natural source of sugar (not refined sugar), ingredients I understand, and, most importantly, I like this energy bar!

Let's recap

So far in this chapter on diet, we haven't even put anything in our mouths. I've talked more about the "state" I'd like you to be in when you eat, the preparation process around eating, and some basic nutrition guidelines from a big-picture perspective. I introduced the importance of providing your body with the essential building blocks it needs to support the formation of neurotransmitters. In the next chapter, I'll delve into the specifics of *what* to eat.

STEPS FOR HEALTHY EATING

....

1. Cook real food.
2. Breathe.
3. Chew.
4. Relax.

And remember: No multitasking while eating!

---

(11)

Diet and Supplements—
You Are What You Eat, Part 2

"Every moment is an opportunity to start anew."
DR. CHRIS

OR MENTAL WELL-BEING and weight management, there are many theories about what to eat and what not to eat. It is my intention to make this clear and easy for you. Simply put, you need to ensure your diet incorporates all the essential macromolecules, or nutritional building blocks, that your body requires to make the neurotransmitters and hormones that are responsible for a balanced mood. These include:

- Essential amino acids involved in neurotransmitter formation: tryptophan for serotonin and phenylalanine for dopamine
- Essential fats involved in both neurotransmitter and hormone formation: omega 3 and omega 6
- Nutrients involved in neurotransmitter formation: vitamin B3, vitamin B6, magnesium, vitamin C, vitamin D, folate, iron, riboflavin and zinc

Serotonin recap

Food has a significant influence on the brain's behaviour. A poor diet, especially one high in junk food, is a common cause of mental dis-ease.

The levels of neurotransmitters are controlled by what we eat. As mentioned in Chapter 10, one very important neurotransmitter is serotonin, as it plays a role in mood, sleep and appetite. Low levels of serotonin may result from diets too high in simple sugars/carbohydrates (e.g., white sugar, white flour, sweets, processed foods), which leads to depression, anxiety, binge eating and sleep disturbances. Diets high in complex carbohydrates (e.g., vegetables, whole grains, legumes and beans), on the other hand, help to increase serotonin and elevate mood.

Serotonin is derived from the essential amino acid tryptophan. By increasing tryptophan-containing foods, we can increase the amount of serotonin made in the brain. I struggled with my mental health for more than 15 years, and in that time, not one doctor ever asked me what I was eating. When I was in my second year studying naturopathic medicine, we had to analyze our diets for a nutrition assignment. I was shocked to discover that the only essential amino acid in which I was deficient was tryptophan. This was one of the reasons my mental health improved when I began supplementing my diet with the vitamins and minerals prescribed by Dr. Hoffer: the tryptophan pathway in my body was being supported.

Therapeutic foods

In general, eat a diet that is high in raw fruits and vegetables, whole grains (e.g., brown rice, oats, millet), raw nuts and seeds, and legumes (e.g., chick peas, kidney beans, peas, lentils). Such a diet will ensure adequate amounts of complex carbohydrates to increase serotonin levels in the brain. It is very difficult to meet your vitamin D requirements from food sources, so supplementation is important. Try to emphasize:

- **Foods high in essential fatty acids:** including raw nuts, seeds, vegetable oils (avocado, coconut, safflower, walnut, sunflower), evening primrose oil, flaxseed oil, camelina oil and black currant oil (essential fatty acids are needed for normal brain function)

- **Foods rich in vitamin B6 & B3:** including 100% bran cereal, millet, brown rice, watermelon, bananas, avocado, chicken, turkey, rainbow trout, sunflower seeds, halibut, sweet potato, potato, tuna, broccoli, walnuts, oat bran, feta cheese, salmon, beans (e.g., chickpeas, kidney beans, lentils, lima beans, and pinto beans)

- **Foods high in tryptophan:** including turkey, tuna, salmon (wild), cashews, halibut, shrimp, oatmeal flakes, cottage cheese, pork, avocado, wheat germ, eggs, collards, spinach, raisins, yogourt, chicken, sweet potato

- **Foods high in vitamin C:** including peppers (red, yellow, green), broccoli, red cabbage, Brussels sprouts, kohlrabi, snow peas, cauliflower, kale, rapini, bok choy, sweet potato, turnip greens, tomato, acerola berries, guava, papaya, kiwi, orange, lychee, strawberries, pineapple, grapefruit, cantaloupe, honeydew melon, mango, berries (raspberries, blueberries, blackberries), watermelon

- **Foods high in zinc:** including oysters, beef, wheat germ, turkey (dark meat), Swiss chard, lima beans, potatoes, rolled oats, mustard greens, pumpkin seeds, soybeans, tuna, kidney beans, wild rice, peas, leeks, lentils, cashews, sunflower seeds, lima beans, pecans, tahini (sesame butter), peanuts

- **Foods high in magnesium:** including soybean flour, buckwheat flour, soybeans, tofu, rye, dried figs, black-eyed peas, Swiss chard, almonds, cashews, brown rice, kidney beans, filberts, lima beans, halibut, Brazil nuts, pecans, kelp, peanuts, walnuts, banana, beet greens, avocado, potato, oat bran, navy beans, watermelon, acorn squash, millet, cocoa powder, blackstrap molasses, sweet potato, oatmeal, wheat bran, okra, kiwi, spinach, chickpeas, peas, winter squash, collards

- **Foods high in vitamin B12:** including beef, clams, salmon, lamb, lobster, beef liver, tuna, milk, halibut, eggs, chicken (vitamin B12 is generally not present in plant foods, but fortified breakfast cereals and milks are a source of vitamin B12 for vegans and vegetarians)

- **Liver-cleansing foods:** including beets, carrots, artichokes, lemons, parsnips, dandelion greens, watercress, burdock root

Foods to avoid

- **Aspartame and other artificial sweeteners** (e.g., NutraSweet, Equal, Splenda). These are found in many diet sodas and sugar-free gums. Aspartame can block the formation of serotonin and cause headaches, insomnia and depression in individuals who are already serotonin-deprived.

- Any foods known or suspected to trigger your allergies or sensitivities.

- **Alcohol, caffeine (including coffee and black tea) and processed foods.** Caffeine can play a strong role in depression for some individuals. Intake of caffeine should not exceed 150 milligrams per day. Note that one cup of brewed coffee has 95 to 150 milligrams of caffeine and one cup of tea has up to 70 milligrams of caffeine. The harmful effects of caffeine are discussed further in Chapter 12.

- **Foods high in saturated fats:** fatty beef/hamburger, lamb, pork, poultry with skin, tallow, lard, cream, butter, cheese, French fries or other fried foods. Such foods lead to sluggishness, slow thinking, fatigue and eventually poor circulation (especially to the brain).

- **Sugar and excessive amounts of simple carbohydrates:** including "good" sweeteners, such as honey, agave, molasses and fruit juice. These simple carbohydrates and refined sugars initially increase energy, but this is quickly followed by fatigue and depression. Sugar also depletes the body of B vitamins and magnesium, which are crucial to the production of serotonin. Note: Stevia (a concentrated natural sweetener derived from a South American shrub) is an acceptable substitute available at health food stores.

- **Wheat and foods containing wheat.** Wheat gluten has been linked to depressive disorders.

In the Appendix, you will find a Mental Health Diet that includes a two-week menu plan and recipes to support optimal mental well-being. If your diet currently consists of the following ...

BREAKFAST: Muffin and coffee with cream and sugar
LUNCH: Hamburger, large fries and pop (fast food)
DINNER: Spaghetti and meatballs

... then you may find the Mental Health Diet, as well as the suggestions about foods to avoid, overwhelming. After my first visit to a naturopathic doctor, I was told I should cut out wheat, dairy, sugar, chocolate, tomatoes and eggs. I found myself wondering, "What's left to eat?" This was in the mid-1990s, long before there was any information about the negative effects of wheat and when gluten-free products were practically non-existent in mainstream grocery stores. I also didn't know what quinoa was, let alone how to pronounce, spell or cook it.

At that time, breakfast was typically a piece of fruit. I usually ate out for lunch—sometimes fast food or a healthier meal if I was taken out for lunch by a supplier. And dinner was either a can of soup or a potato cooked in the microwave with grated cheddar cheese and salsa on top. I lived in my apartment for eight years and rarely used my oven. When I got married, I had never cooked a turkey or a roast, given my vegetarian background and lack of interest in cooking. Simply put, I didn't know how to cook, and I was too busy climbing the corporate ladder to care.

Guidelines for eating well

So, I hear you. I get it. I've been there. And my suggestion is to incorporate one meal or snack per day from the Mental Health Diet. Cooking is easy. You've got this. It doesn't have to be complicated. Start by focusing on the positive suggestions around food, such as increasing tryptophan-forming foods or foods high in essential fatty acids, and don't worry as much about what to avoid. In time, your good food choices will push out the "bad" ones. I keep my meals simple: a protein (chicken, turkey or wild fish), a complex carbohydrate (brown rice or quinoa), and lots of vegetables. The key is to start somewhere that feels possible for you. What is not an option is doing nothing. Get started by introducing meals from the Mental Health Diet, as well as incorporating one or more of the suggestions below.

1. **Eat a good breakfast and don't skip meals:** It is important to have a small amount of protein (nuts, avocado, eggs or yogourt) and a variety of fruits, vegetables and hearty whole grains for breakfast to carry you through until lunch. If you skip a meal, you increase the likelihood that you will be excessively hungry later in the day and more likely to eat too much of the "wrong" type of food. A great place to start is by incorporating the breakfast recipes outlined in the Mental Health Diet (see the Appendix).

2. **Eat slowly:** Take at least 20 minutes to eat a meal, as it takes this long for your stomach to send the "full" message to your brain. By rushing your meals, you can eat too much before you realize you are satisfied.

3. **Shop smart:** Nutritious foods are found around the perimeters of grocery stores, not in boxes in the food aisles.

4. **Do not go shopping when you are hungry.** You're more likely to give in to the temptation to buy things you know you shouldn't eat.

5. **Avoid buying junk food** and other foods that are high in fat, sugar or salt.

6. **Learn to read labels.** Avoid items with the following words in the ingredients list: refined, sugar, agave, glucose, high-fructose corn syrup, sucrose, hydrogenated, sugar alcohol (sorbitol, xylitol, mannitol) and artificial sweetener (saccharin, aspartame, NutraSweet, Equal, Splenda).

7. **Prepare for times of weakness:** Recognize times or events that signal you to eat something you shouldn't, such as an argument, a hard day at work, talking on the phone, watching TV, or just being bored. Plan activities for these situations that don't involve poor food choices, such as exercising, taking a long bath, journalling, or reading a good book.

8. **Be your own best friend:** If your friend makes a mistake, you don't call them a failure or tell them to give up. Cut yourself the same slack: If you stray from your eating plan, don't be hard on yourself. Treat each lapse as temporary, not as a sign of failure. Simply resume your program and don't look back. You can make a new choice with each bite. If you find yourself knee-deep in an ice-cream container, remember to ask yourself with each bite if you want to continue. If the answer is no and you continue eating, you may need further support to recognize why you cross this boundary with yourself.

9. **Call "treats" what they are: dead-energy foods with no vitality.** The food industry has manipulated the levels of fat, sugar and salt in their products so that we will become addicted to them. They aren't interested in your health and well-being; they are interested in selling a product and making money. That is why it is important to recognize that the types of foods we commonly refer to as "treats" aren't actually treats to our biochemistry. Foods such as ice cream, cake, cookies, chocolate, pop, Slurpees, chips, cheezies and so on contribute to chaos in our bodies from a blood sugar perspective instead of calmness. It is best if we refer to these foods as either salt-, fat- or sugar-laden, dead-energy foods with no vitality. Does this sound appetizing? Is this really what you want to be eating? Remember that sugar is a highly addictive substance. To eliminate it from your life,

you have to wean off it and develop a healthier relationship with it. Start by cutting portion sizes in half, skipping dessert most nights, and substituting fresh fruit for highly processed sugary snacks. Remember that sugar is not a treat for your body. See Chapter 13 for more information on sugar.

10. **Drink plenty of water (filtered, with minerals remaining):** Water flushes toxins from your body and helps keep your appetite under control. The minimum amount we need per day is half our body weight (in pounds) in ounces. For example, a 160-pound individual needs to consume a minimum of 80 ounces, which is equivalent to 2.5 litres. I keep a large water bottle beside my bed, and the first thing I do when my feet hit the floor in the morning is drink as much water as I can. It is best to drink more water during the day so you don't disrupt your sleep at night by going to the bathroom. Ideally, to avoid exposure to harmful endocrine disruptors, store your water in glass or stainless steel containers instead of plastic.

Using supplements wisely

While diet is extremely important, it is often difficult to get from food the medicinal doses of the essential nutrients we need to support the formation of neurotransmitters and hormones. This is because the quality of our soil is not what it used to be and the demands for nutrients are high, as every cell in our body requires them. For example, vitamin C is a nutrient required to support the conversion of tryptophan to serotonin, and the minimum recommended dose is 2,000 milligrams per day. Since one orange contains approximately 80 milligrams of vitamin C, you would have to eat 25 oranges per day to meet this requirement from food. Since many people have poor diets, supplements are necessary building blocks to recovery while the dietary changes are being made. Personally, I feel it is important to eat the right foods as cleanly as possible, in addition to taking supplements. When you eat clean and avoid pesticides, you reduce the possibility that chemicals used in the food manufacturing process will end up as bouncers blocking the receptors in your brain.

My philosophy with supplements and pharmaceuticals is: minimum dose for maximum benefit for the shortest duration. At the start of treatment, higher doses are often required. Once we see improvement, medication levels may need to be adjusted to maintain health. I explain that it takes a lot of fuel to get an airplane off the ground (i.e., higher doses), but once it gets to cruising altitude (i.e., feeling better), then you can decrease the amount of fuel needed to reach your destination. I provide patients with customized advice on dosages, but here I am providing general guidelines since it's difficult for me to recommend the right dose of a nutrient for you without taking your case. I would encourage you to consult with a naturopathic doctor if you need further guidance. The common nutrients that are prescribed in naturopathic medicine to support mental health include: the B vitamins (B6, B3, B5, B12, B1, B2), folic acid, vitamin C, zinc, magnesium, iron, omega 3s and vitamin D. Also, there are many nutrients required for the proper functioning of hormones (i.e., adrenals, thyroid), which is why it is best to consult with a naturopathic doctor, who can make individualized recommendations.

In terms of supplementation, there are a few common mistakes that people make.

1. **They believe diet is enough and supplements aren't necessary.** For many health conditions, you need more nutrients than the recommended daily allowance (RDA) suggests. Keep in mind that the RDA is set at recommended levels for *healthy* individuals and may not be enough if you have a health concern (e.g., depression, anxiety, hormone imbalances, fatigue, high blood pressure). Also, we are exposed to a barrage of potentially harmful chemicals daily; therefore, we require more nutrients to support our bodies' ability to detoxify and eliminate them.

2. **They take the wrong form of a nutrient.** Many nutrients come in different forms, and some are better than others. When it comes to minerals, some inhibit absorption of others, and imbalanced ratios in the body can contribute to mental health conditions, such as too much copper creating a zinc deficiency. This is why it is best to see a naturopathic doctor, who can help navigate the nutrient highway for you. These are the correct forms of nutrients to be discussing with your naturopathic doctor if you have a mental health concern:

   • **Folic acid/folate:** It is commonly assumed that these words are interchangeable, but there is an important difference. Folic acid is a synthetic derivative that must be converted in the body to the natural active form of folate known as 5-methyltetrahydrofolate

(5MTHF). Many people are unable to make these conversion steps, which is why supplementing with 5MTHF is recommended.

- **Vitamin B12:** This vitamin is found in three forms: cyanocobalamin, hydroxycobalamin and methylcobalamin. The most absorbable and best-utilized form is methylcobalamin.

- **Vitamin B3:** There are three forms of vitamin B3: niacin (nicotinic acid), niacinamide (nicotinamide) and inositol hexanicotinate. For mental health, niacin and niacinamide are the preferred forms. In higher doses (greater than 50 milligrams), niacin can cause a flush reaction. This is when the skin becomes red and itchy and you may have a burning or tingling sensation. Since many find it uncomfortable, the non-flushing form of niacin, niacinamide, is often prescribed. If high doses of niacin are taken over a long period of time, liver enzymes can become elevated, so these need to be monitored.

- **Vitamin B6:** The best-utilized form for anxiety and depression is pyridoxal 5'phosphate.

- **Magnesium and iron:** The best-utilized form for anxiety and depression is the bisglycinate form.

- **Zinc:** The best-utilized forms for depression and anxiety are either zinc citrate or picolinate.

- **Omega 3s:** There are three types of omega 3s: alpha linoleic acid (ALA), eicosapentaenoic acid (EPA) and docosahexaenoic acid (DHA). Although ALA can serve as the precursor for EPA and DHA synthesis, this pathway is limited in its capacity and varies between individuals. With mental health conditions, supplementation of EPA and DHA is recommended in a minimum 2:1 ratio of EPA:DHA.

3. **They take the wrong dose of a nutrient.** It is common for patients to dismiss a nutrient as ineffective. When I ask about the dose they were taking, most of the time, it was too low. There is an anti-vitamin spin to most media reports on vitamin research, and the message that gets promoted is that vitamin therapy does not work. This is nonsense. There are thousands of nutritional research studies that provide evidence that vitamins can help prevent and treat serious diseases, including mental illness and heart disease, when supplied in high

enough doses. This is the key: the correct dose is required. Says cardiologist Thomas Levy, MD: "The three most important considerations in effective vitamin C therapy are dose, dose, and dose. If you don't take enough, you won't get the desired effects."

4. **They take supplements with poor-quality non-medicinal ingredients.** The other day a patient brought in a garlic pill for me to assess. One of the ingredients listed on the label was hydrogenated oil. I was shocked! With all the bad press about the dangers of hydrogenated oil and trans fats, why would it be in a supplement? Yet, there it was. It is important to read labels—particularly the list of non-medicinal ingredients, of which there should be no more than five. To determine whether a hard tablet supplement you are taking contains fillers and sugars, place them on a baking sheet covered in tinfoil and bake for 15 min at 350 F. The tablets should change colour mildly and/or look "baked," as food would. Many poor-quality products burn into a black mass because of the fillers and sugars used in manufacturing.

5. **They take poor-quality supplements that are hard to absorb.** Another concern with supplements is whether you are absorbing the nutrients you are ingesting. To do that, you have to be able to break the supplement down. Naturopathic doctors prescribe professional-quality supplements that are either liquid, powder- or vegetable-capsule-based. We rarely prescribe hard tablets because they are difficult to break down. To determine if you are absorbing a hard tablet supplement, put it into a quarter cup of vinegar. It should dissolve within a half hour, as vinegar approximates the acidity of your stomach. If it doesn't dissolve, it is unlikely you are breaking it down properly to assimilate the essential nutrients it contains.

Like my mom keeps telling me: If you buy a cheap pair of shoes, you will be replacing them next year. However, spend a little more money for a quality pair and it will last you for years. I can attest to this because I still own the same pair of black dress shoes that I had in my banking career days in the 1990s. The same can be said about supplements: You pay for what you get, and when it comes to your body, you want to make sure you are supplementing with the right nutrients. It's important that you get the right form and dose of a nutrient. This is why it is best to consult with a naturopathic doctor.

While I have focused on supplements in this section, it is important to note that there are many amazing plants with therapeutic benefits in the treatment of mental health conditions. These include St. John's wort, oats, borage, lemon balm, catnip, lavender and passionflower, to name a few. It is best to be under the care of a naturopathic doctor who is trained in herbs, homeopathics and supplements, as well as pharmaceutical medications, when taking these.

(12)

Sugar, Caffeine and Weight

*"Your relationship with food reflects the relationship you have
with yourself. Do you like what you see?"*

DR. CHRIS

D O YOU FIND you can't get through the day without a sugary snack?
You may be one of many people who are "addicted" to sugar. Signs
of sugar addiction include irritability, headaches, mood swings
and insomnia. Sugar addiction is, in part, a by-product of sugar's purity.
The body is not suited to accommodating this level of refinement. Simple sugars—found in white table sugar, corn syrup, fructose, white flour
or any other super-refined carbohydrates—are refined to the point that
digestion is practically superfluous.

The problem with sugar

When you consume simple sugars, they pass quickly into the bloodstream.
Your blood sugar levels skyrocket, and you experience a lift in energy. But
that feeling of increased energy and mental alertness is temporary. As
most of us can confirm, sugar highs lead to sugar crashes. And when that
buzz wears off, the body cries out for more sugar. This dangerous blood
sugar roller-coaster ride sets people up for future health disease, such as
obesity, type 2 diabetes and cardiovascular disease. Simply providing the
body with more sugar does not address the root problem.

Sugar is the one substance that I have a bumpy, rocky, rickety relationship with. I can eliminate it for months at a time, and then something happens, such as a birthday or a chocolate occasion (Valentine's Day, Easter, Halloween, Christmas), and I have one piece, and the next thing you know, I am craving it again and having a hard time resisting it.

Some of the underlying causes for sugar cravings are low endorphin levels, hypoglycemia, hormone imbalances, candida overgrowth and nutritional deficiencies. To determine if candida could be playing a role in your health, complete the Candida Questionnaire.

CANDIDA QUESTIONNAIRE

Candida may be playing a role in your mental health if you have many of the following symptoms. Count your major symptoms first, then your other symptoms, and add your scores.

(A) HISTORY

For each "yes" answer, circle the point total and record your score at the end of this section.

Point Score

1. Have you ever taken tetracycline, erythromycin or any other antibiotic for 1 month or longer to treat acne?   **25**
2. Have you, at any time in your life, taken other "broad spectrum" antibiotics for respiratory, urinary or other infections (for 2 months or more, or in shorter courses 4 times in a 1-year period)?   **20**
3. Have you ever taken a broad spectrum antibiotic— even a single course?   **6**
4. Have you, at any time in your life, been bothered by persistent vaginitis, prostatitis or other problems affecting your reproductive organs?   **25**
5. Have you been pregnant...
   2 or more times?   **5**
   1 time?   **3**
6. Have you taken birth control pills...
   For more than 2 years?   **15**
   For 6 months to 2 years?   **8**

7.   Have you taken prednisone or any other cortisone-type drugs
     For more than 2 weeks?   **15**
     For 2 weeks or less?   **6**
8.   Does exposure to perfume, insecticides or other chemicals provoke...
     Moderate to severe symptoms?   **20**
     Mild symptoms?   **5**
9.   Are your symptoms worse on a damp, muggy days or in mouldy
     places?   **20**
10. Have you had athlete's foot, ring worm, "jock itch" or other chronic
     fungus infections of the skin or nails? Have such infections been...
     Severe or persistent?   **20**
     Mild to moderate?   **10**
11. Do you crave sugar?   **10**
12. Do you crave breads?   **10**
13. Do you crave alcoholic beverages?   **10**
14. Does tobacco smoke *really* bother you?   **10**

TOTAL SCORE (A): _____

(B) MAJOR SYMPTOMS

For each of your symptoms, enter the appropriate figure in the Point Score
column:

If a symptom is:

Occasional or mild .... 3 **pts.**
Frequent and/or moderately severe .... 6 **pts.**
Severe and/or disabling .... 9 **pts.**

Record total score at the end of this section.

Point Score
1.   Fatigue or lethargy _____
2.   Feeling of being "drained" _____
3.   Poor memory _____
4.   Feeling "spacey" or "unreal" _____
5.   Depression _____
6.   Numbness, burning or tingling _____
7.   Muscles aches _____

8. Muscle weakness or paralysis _____
9. Pain and/or swelling in joints _____
10. Abdominal pain _____
11. Constipation _____
12. Diarrhea _____
13. Bloating _____
14. Troublesome vaginal discharge _____
15. Persistent vaginal burning or itching _____
16. Prostatitis _____
17. Impotence _____
18. Loss of sexual desire _____
19. Endometriosis _____
20. Cramps/other menstrual problems _____
21. Premenstrual tension _____
22. Spots in front of the eyes _____
23. Erratic vision _____

TOTAL SCORE (B): _____

(C) OTHER SYMPTOMS

For each of your symptoms, enter the appropriate figure in the Point Score column:

If a symptom is:

Occasional or mild ....1 pts.
Frequent and/or moderately severe ....2 pts.
Severe and/or disabling ....3 pts.

Record total score at the end of this section.

Point Score
1. Drowsiness _____
2. Irritability or jitteriness _____
3. Poor coordination _____
4. Inability to concentrate _____
5. Frequent mood swings _____
6. Headache _____
7. Dizziness/loss of balance _____

8. Pressure above ears/"head swelling" _____
9. Itching _____
10. Other rashes _____
11. Heartburn _____
12. Indigestion _____
13. Belching and intestinal gas _____
14. Mucous in stools _____
15. Hemorrhoids _____
16. Dry mouth _____
17. Rash or blisters in mouth _____
18. Bad breath _____
19. Joint swelling or arthritis _____
20. Congestion _____
21. Postnasal drip _____
22. Nasal itching _____
23. Sore throat or dry throat _____
24. Cough _____
25. Pain or tightness in chest _____
26. Wheezing or shortness of breath _____
27. Urgency or urinary frequency _____
28. Burning on urination _____
29. Failing vision _____
30. Burning or tearing eyes _____
31. Recurrent infection or fluid in ears _____
32. Ear pain or deafness _____

TOTAL SCORE (C) _____

ADD TOTAL SCORE (B) _____

ADD TOTAL SCORE (A) _____

GRAND TOTAL SCORE _____

The Grand Total Score will help you and your physician decide if your health problems are yeast connected. Scores in women will run higher, as seven items in the questionnaire apply exclusively to women while only two apply exclusively to men.

Yeast-connected health problems are almost certainly present in women with scores over 180, and in men with scores over 140. With scores of less than 60 in women and 40 in men, yeast is less apt to cause health problems.

Some of the factors that make it more likely for people to develop a problem with yeast are poor nutrition and impaired immunity. If you suspect you may have a candida problem, please see your naturopathic doctor.

"Candida Questionnaire and Score Sheet" from The Yeast Connection: A Medical Breakthrough by William G. Crook, copyright © 1983, 1984, 1985, 1986 by William G. Crook, M.D. Used by permission of Random House, an imprint and division of Penguin Random House LLC. All rights reserved.

Sugar is also an antidepressant of sorts. Eating it triggers the release of the brain chemical serotonin, which elevates mood and alleviates depression. Sugar cravings are often a misguided attempt by the body to elevate mood by increasing serotonin levels. The good news is that there are many other foods that increase serotonin levels without setting you up for long-term health consequences.

It's best to withdraw from sugar gradually, as quitting cold turkey can lead to restlessness, nervousness, headaches and depression. It is also important to note that sugar negatively affects liver and immune function, creating the perfect terrain for viral, bacterial or fungal "bugs" to take hold. If you are reading this and are currently depressed, my recommendation is not to quit sugar immediately, given that sugar withdrawal can result in increased levels of depression. A first step to get off the blood sugar roller-coaster is to drink more water and increase the amount of complex carbohydrates (vegetables, whole grains and legumes) and protein (tryptophan foods) in your diet. These take longer to digest, so your blood sugar level increases slowly and declines gradually. The best time to reduce your sugar intake is when you are no longer feeling depressed.

Here are some suggestions to help you break up with sugar:

1. **Watch documentaries on sugar.** *Fed Up, Sugar Coated, Hungry for Change, The Secrets of Sugar* and *Fat, Sick and Nearly Dead* will increase your awareness and provide more incentive to decrease how much sugar you eat.

2. **Remember your math.** On food labels, sugar is quoted in grams. But what does this really mean? I find it helpful to remember that 4 grams of sugar is equal to 1 teaspoon. This gives me a better visual when I am

reading labels. For example, I was eating organic vanilla flavoured yogourt that contained 24 grams of sugar per half-cup serving. This is the equivalent of 6 teaspoons of sugar, which is a lot! In this case, it is better to buy plain yogourt and mix in a quarter-cup of fresh fruit.

3.   **Eat within your limits.** As you are decreasing the amount of sugar in your diet, try to determine your average daily consumption by keeping a diet diary. From there, you can make changes. Aim to have one or two teaspoons less of sugar per day until it is eliminated from your diet.

4.   **Avoid processed junk foods.** Sugar is an addictive substance that has a powerful influence on your brain. Sugar stimulates a region of your brain called the nucleus accumbens, causing it to produce dopamine, the pleasure neurotransmitter. Soon dopamine levels drop and we start to feel flat, or a bit "down." We crave the pleasant, feel-good feeling again, so we reach for sugar—the cycle of addiction has begun. The best thing you can do to help break this cycle is avoid processed junk food that is high in sugar.

5.   **Boost your serotonin.** Serotonin, also known as "the happiness hormone," can be raised through a naturally low-glycemic diet (such as the Mental Health Diet in the Appendix), daily exercise and plenty of deep, restful sleep. When you have enough serotonin, you are less likely to crave sugar.

6.   **Use stevia to satisfy your sweet tooth.** The all-natural sweetener stevia has zero calories and does not raise blood sugar levels despite being 300 times sweeter than sugar. If you have sugar cravings and want to satisfy your sweet tooth, stevia is a safe bet. Stevia comes in both liquid and powder form and is available in most grocery and health food stores.

7.   **Stay hydrated with water.** You may sometimes think your body is asking for sugar when in fact it's dehydrated and craving water. Remember the rule of thumb with water is to drink half your body weight (in pounds) in ounces. Many people complain about the taste of water, so try this simple, delicious cravings-buster lemonade: to one cup of water, add the juice of half a lemon and five drops of stevia. You could also try a warm cup of raspberry tea, sweetened with stevia, after your meal. This satisfies your sweet tooth and you won't want dessert.

8. **Stabilize your blood sugar levels.** Eat complex carbohydrates and good fats at every meal to sustain your blood sugar levels. Include a gluten-free grain, such as quinoa, millet, buckwheat or amaranth, in your evening meal. If you do this, your body will produce more serotonin, you'll feel happier and you'll sleep much better at night.

9. **Have plenty of greens.** Loaded with nutrition, greens boost your energy and help reduce cravings for sugar and processed foods. Experiment with making juices using a combination of lemon, pear and/or apple and the following greens: celery, cucumber, kale, spinach and/or parsley. To reduce your exposure to pesticides used in the growing process, it is best to eat organic forms of apples, cucumbers and celery. (See the Dirty Dozen and Clean Fifteen lists in Chapter 16, which outline the foods most and least sprayed with pesticides.)

10. **Eat more seaweed.** Loaded with vitamins and minerals, seaweed is a great addition to salads and meals. Seaweed is rich in minerals and helps restore mineral levels that can be depleted by sugar. Seaweed examples are dulse, kelp, wakame, arame and nori. Sprinkle dulse flakes on your salad or on an avocado. Add seaweed to your soups for a rich, salty mineral flavour.

11. **Consume more fermented foods and drinks.** These are an important way to reduce or even eliminate sugar cravings. Try fermented kefir, sauerkraut, kimchi, kombucha and natural plain yogourt. You will be amazed at how the sour taste of fermented foods and drinks quells the desire for sugar and processed foods.

12. **Use fresh fruit as a healthy sugar substitute.** Summer is such a great time to incorporate healthy fruit into your diet. Remind yourself what sugary, processed foods really are: dead-energy food with no vitality. Compare that with a strawberry that is bursting with flavour, or a slice of juicy watermelon. Enjoy the vitality of fresh fruit and you will kick your craving for unhealthy, sugary foods.

13. **Learn meditation and stress-reduction techniques.** Meditation can help ward off cravings by helping to reduce stress. Stress creates the hormone cortisol, which increases blood sugar levels. This is a vicious cycle that contributes to hormone imbalances and creates sugar cravings. Try exercise, yoga or meditation before or after work to calm your body and mind.

14. **Try the Emotional Freedom Technique (EFT).** If you're looking to shift the desire for sugar, lose weight, stop a habit of bingeing or eliminate any addiction, you owe it to yourself to learn about EFT. EFT is an easy tool that anyone can learn in minutes. You simply tap on emotional acupressure points on your body while repeating key statements that help shift your body, mind and habits. For more information, see Nick Ortner's book *The Tapping Solution*.

The problem with caffeine

Is coffee part of your morning routine? Are you convinced it's good for you? Everything in moderation, right? Maybe not in this case.

Since the explosion of Starbucks, Tim Hortons and Second Cup, the popularity of coffee has led people to turn a blind eye to the harmful health effects of caffeine. But the dangers are clear, and it is hard to refute the fact that caffeine is an addictive substance that causes a range of symptoms.

I am often met with resistance when I ask people to eliminate caffeine (in all forms) from their diet. However, once I explain the harmful effects of caffeine and the benefits of reducing their intake or eliminating it entirely, compliance increases. A colleague uses this analogy to explain caffeine's effects on the body:

Imagine you have a pair of soaked sponges. They are so full that the minute you pick them up, they spill over with excess water. These are your healthy adrenal glands that are spilling over with energy-producing, stress-regulating hormones, such as cortisol. With each event in your life, you start to squeeze the sponges little by little:

- Teenage years and parties
- University stress/cramming for exams
- College parties
- Finding a job after graduation
- Starting a career
- Buying a car
- Moving and buying a home
- Dating
- Planning a wedding and honeymoon

- Work promotions
- Having a child
- Having another child
- Divorce
- Death of a loved one
- Caring for aging parents
- Moving, etc.

If you don't take time to recharge your batteries, or in this case refill your sponges, they will slowly start to dry out. When daily tasks become major stressors and you fall into a reactive mindset, caffeine can save the day. Caffeine does a fantastic job at stimulating your adrenal glands to produce more stress-regulating hormones. Unfortunately, when you're in survival mode, you are often not taking the time to rest and eat properly and nourish your adrenals—so your sponges dry out even more. Instead of one cup of coffee in the morning, you now need three. Eventually, you wring out the last few drops of cortisol and reach "adrenal fatigue." Your body is no longer able to function properly, and you can physically collapse. This is often seen after someone finishes a big project, goes out to celebrate and within days finds themselves sick.

It's important to recognize that caffeine is an addictive substance and that it can be a slippery slope to addiction. A few questions to ask yourself are:

1. Why do you need caffeine? Is it a pick-me-up because you're tired? If so, have you addressed why you're so tired? If you have problems sleeping, is it possible that caffeine is disturbing your sleep?
2. If you go without caffeine, do you experience withdrawal symptoms?

I am asking these questions to help you think about your behaviour. My goal as a health care provider is to assess patients' diets to see if what they are consuming daily is contributing to their health issues or supporting vitality. It's important to remember that everything that passes into your body *informs* your body. You are made of nutritional building blocks, such as water, vitamins, minerals, protein and fats. As mentioned, some of these nutrients are essential. This means that we can't make them ourselves, and we must get them from our diet. If we don't, we will be deficient.

Let's look at the list of potential side effects from overuse of caffeine:

1. **Negative influence on vitamins and minerals**
   - Caffeine's diuretic effect depletes important minerals (calcium, magnesium, potassium, zinc, iron) and vitamins (vitamin B1, vitamin C).

   - Coffee reduces your ability to absorb iron, calcium and vitamin D, especially when you drink it with food. These nutrients are extremely important, as deficiencies can lead to mental health concerns, osteoporosis and anemia.

   - In children and adolescents, caffeinated drinks interfere with essential minerals needed for growth and development.

2. **Gastrointestinal irritation**
   - As little as one cup of coffee stimulates acid secretion in the stomach for more than an hour in a healthy individual. In someone with an ulcer, the effect is greater and lasts more than two hours.

   - Long-term use of caffeine can play a role in ulcer formation. It can aggravate an existing ulcer and interfere with the healing process.

   - Overusing caffeine can also cause diarrhea by relaxing the smooth muscle in the colon. This laxative effect can also make your large colon dependent on caffeine for bowel movements. This gives many the illusion that they have healthy bowel function when they are using a stimulant every day to induce a bowel movement.

3. **Cardiovascular system effects**
   - Caffeine raises your blood pressure. Hypertension is a risk factor in atherosclerosis and heart disease.

   - Caffeine increases blood levels of cholesterol and triglycerides, which are risk factors in cardiovascular disease.

   - Heart rhythm disturbances and arrhythmias can occur with caffeine consumption. Disturbances include an increased heart rate and excitability of the heart nerve conduction system, leading to both palpitations and extra beats.

   - Caffeine also increases norepinephrine secretion, causing constriction of the arteries and leading to restricted blood flow.

   - Due to the way caffeine stimulates the cardiovascular system, it seems reasonable to assume that long-term consumption of four to five cups of coffee per day can increase the incidence of heart attacks (myocardial infarction).

- The cardiovascular effects of caffeine are often labelled as anxiety when they are really a symptom of having too much of the substance.

4. **Central nervous system effects**
   - Caffeine is a central nervous system stimulant. It works by blocking the effects of adenosine, which is a substance created in the brain. Adenosine binds to receptors and slows down nerve cells. This causes drowsiness and blood vessels to increase in diameter to let more oxygen in during sleep. Caffeine has a similar shape to adenosine and binds to its receptors, but it has a stimulating effect and speeds up nerve cells, increasing energy.

   - Common central nervous system side effects of caffeine use include: nervousness, irritability, insomnia, "restless legs," dizziness, headaches and fatigue. Psychological symptoms of depression, general anxiety or panic attacks may also occur. Hyperactivity and bed wetting may develop in children who consume caffeine.

   - Caffeine may make you more likely to become addicted to something else. Experiments with animals show that when coffee is added to the diet, animals voluntarily drink more alcohol than the amount they would otherwise consume.

   - Caffeine enters the blood, and can start causing effects 15 minutes after it is consumed. It then takes about six hours for one-half of the caffeine to be eliminated.

5. **Exhausting effects**
   - Caffeine increases blood sugar levels (especially when sweetened) by stimulating the adrenal glands. Over time, both stress, caffeine and sugar consumption combine to weaken adrenal function, resulting in fatigue. People turn to coffee for that morning pick-me-up since caffeine can override this fatigue by stimulating the adrenals. The problem is that over time, this habit contributes to chronic fatigue, adrenal exhaustion and subsequent inability to handle stress and sugar intake. As such, adrenal exhaustion/stress/fatigue/hypoglycemia syndromes are associated with caffeine use.

6. **Cancer-causing effects**
   - The incidence of bladder, prostate, ovarian, stomach and pancreatic cancers increases with caffeine use.
   - The risk of ovarian cancer is increased in women with long-term coffee intake of more than five cups per day.
   - Pancreatic cancer has also been observed to occur more frequently with increased coffee use (more than three cups per day).
   - Prostate enlargement and prostate cancer may also be attributed to increased caffeine intake.
   - There is a higher incidence of stomach cancer with more than five cups of coffee per day.

7. **Other effects**
   - Caffeine is correlated with kidney stones, possibly because of its diuretic effect and of the effects of chemicals used in processing coffee.
   - Fibrocystic breast disease may also be a consequence of caffeine use. There is an increase in the size and number of cysts with caffeine consumption. A reduction/reversal of the condition is experienced when caffeine is eliminated from the diet.

How much is safe?
150 to 300 milligrams per day is thought to be a moderate daily intake and is not linked to any negative health effects.

Decreasing your caffeine intake
- Cut back gradually. Keep a log of how much caffeine you consume (remember to include medications), then gradually decrease coffee by a cup per day.
- Substitute with herbal tea, hot cider or healthy coffee substitutes.
- Ask others to decrease coffee intake with you, as there is strength in numbers.
- Dilute your regular coffee with hot water.
- Brew tea or coffee for less time.
- Change your routines. For example, if you need caffeine in the morning to give you a boost, try a light walk for 20 minutes before reaching for your coffee. Physical activity can greatly increase energy levels.

- Ensure you are drinking the minimum water requirement, which is half your body weight (in pounds) in ounces. For example, if you weigh 180 pounds, your minimum water amount is 90 ounces, or 3 litres. Remember that coffee is a diuretic, so depending on how many cups you are drinking per day, you may need to drink more water.

COMMON SYMPTOMS OF CAFFEINE ABUSE

Agitation	Headache	Irritability
Anxiety/nervousness	Heartburn	Nutritional deficiencies
Bed wetting	Increased blood	Poor concentration
Depression	pressure	Tremors
Diarrhea	Increased cholesterol	Ulcers
Dizziness	& triglycerides	Upset stomach
Fatigue	Increased or irregular	
Gastrointestinal	heart rate	
irritation	Insomnia	

COMMON SYMPTOMS OF CAFFEINE WITHDRAWAL

Anxiety/nervousness	Dizziness	Poor concentration
Apathy	Drowsiness/fatigue	Rapid heart rate
Constipation	Feeling cold	Ringing in the ears
Cramps	Headache	Runny nose
Craving	Insomnia	Shakiness
Depression	Irritability	Vomiting
Digestive upsets	Nausea	

WHICH FOODS CONTAIN CAFFEINE?

FOOD	AMOUNT OF CAFFEINE
Coffee – 1 cup (8 oz.)	95–150 mg
Coffee (decaf) – 1 cup	2–12 mg
Green tea – 1 cup	24–45 mg
Black tea – 1 cup	14–70 mg
Hot chocolate – 1 cup	8 mg
Coke, Mountain Dew, Pepsi – 12 oz. (1 can)	46 mg
Cocoa/chocolate – 50 g	3–63 mg
Yerba maté tea – 1 cup	85 mg
DRUGS Exedrin	65 mg
Anacin	32 mg
Midol	32 mg
Dristan	16 mg

A word on weight

Many people with depression, anxiety and disordered eating or eating disorders are concerned about their weight. Since I have had an eating disorder, my philosophy is to teach patients to have a healthy relationship with food and their bodies that is not based on fad diets. The goal is to get to the point where you enjoy what you eat.

Losing weight is a function of five key areas:

- What you eat
- How you eat

- What is eating you mentally, emotionally and spiritually (i.e., stress levels)
- Physiology
- Exercise

You are what you eat

Recognize that 80% of weight loss is determined by diet and the chemical messaging of your hormones. For a minimum of two meals, your plate needs to look like this: 50% vegetables, 25% complex carbohydrates and 25% lean protein (with healthy fats included in these categories). In most circumstances, however, our plates look the opposite, with protein taking up the most space, then a carbohydrate that is usually simple—such as white rice or potatoes—and it is hit and miss with the vegetables.

In terms of what you are eating, it is important to recognize that many diets consist of too much red meat, saturated fat, sodium and alcohol; such a diet provides less nutrition per calorie consumed than a wholesome diet of natural foods. The decreased consumption of vegetables and complex carbohydrates means a lower intake of vitamins, minerals and fibre. Research has linked many well-known diseases (mental health issues, obesity, cardiovascular disease, kidney disease, diabetes, autoimmune diseases, cancer and behavioural problems) with poor diet. Perhaps you don't consider yourself at risk for developing a serious disease, yet you experience the following symptoms: fatigue, headaches, mood swings, depression, indigestion, constipation, skin problems, menstrual discomfort and weight problems. These symptoms not only interfere with your ability to fully enjoy life, but they are also early warning signs for future problems. Eating a healthy diet, such as the Mental Health Diet outlined in the Appendix, can improve these complaints and protect you against serious disease.

How you eat

How you eat your food is as important as what you are eating. Do you inhale your dinner without even thinking? When you do take a bite, is it "chomp, chomp, swallow"? If so, this is one area you can easily improve. It is very important to chew your food thoroughly. I find that in our "fast food nation," many people forget that the digestive process starts in the kitchen, with the sense of smell when we are cooking our food. Food

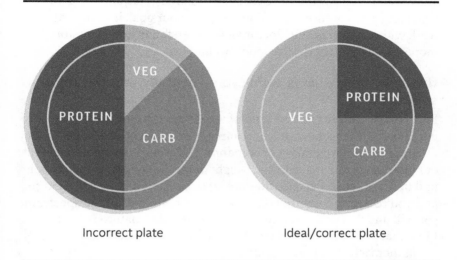

Incorrect plate   Ideal/correct plate

aromas trigger our brains and send the message to our stomach that food is coming. The stomach, in turn, prepares for the arrival of food. When we take the time to chew our food thoroughly, put our forks down between bites and not rush, we are able to adequately process our foods so they can be broken down into the micronutrients that our bodies need to thrive.

The other important component in how we eat relates to the timing of our meals. If we skip breakfast and make dinner our main meal, then we may not be hungry in the morning because we haven't expended any energy sleeping all night. Or if we are constantly snacking throughout the day, then glucose will always be circulating in our veins, making it difficult to lose weight. Both scenarios contribute to hormone imbalances and mismanaged metabolism, which can be addressed by altering our routines.

There is a connection between how we move our bodies and the fuel we provide them with. Think of a car: If your car has a full tank of gas and has been sitting in the garage since the last time you used it, you wouldn't add more fuel to the tank before turning on the engine. If you did, the fuel would have nowhere to go, so it would spill into the environment, polluting and disrupting it. This is what happens when we keep eating and haven't used any fuel. The excess gets stored as fat, and the hormone signalling gets confused. If losing weight is your goal, it is important to work with a naturopathic doctor who understands how to restore hormone signalling patterns to support weight loss.

Understanding what is eating *you*—mentally, emotionally or spiritually

I encourage patients to take note of what emotions they might be "eating" along with that bowl of ice cream—for example, guilt, shame, blame, disappointment, frustration or boredom. These negative emotions affect our physiology and make losing weight more challenging. Many people find they are eating because they are stressed. Or it may be the opposite, and you're eating because you're bored. At both ends of the spectrum, you will find that you are eating unconsciously. As a naturopathic doctor, I feel that an individual's relationship with food reflects how they feel about themselves. It boils down to:

1. Self-esteem or sense of self-love
2. Ability to cope and handle stress
3. Negative self-talk/thought processes and not being in the moment
4. Ability to listen to the messages from your body
5. Shadow and core beliefs about weight that perpetuate any myths you might harbour about losing weight

The first step is to be conscious and present when you eat. Before you reach for a "treat," try to have something healthy first, e.g., fruit or vegetables before you go for the pizza, ice cream, chocolate, candies, doughnuts, a piece of cake or cookies. Celebrate the aliveness and vitality of the food. If, after eating the healthful food first, you still feel you want to have the "treat," then use the five-minute rule from cognitive behavioural therapy. This is where you say to yourself, "I hear you, and in five minutes you can have that sugar-laden, dead-energy food with no vitality." Then wait for five minutes (set the timer if you like) and check in with yourself when the time is up. Most likely, you'll find that the moment has passed and you have moved on. But if after five minutes, you still feel you want to have the "treat," do so. The intention is to break the pattern of resistance. Remember that it is important to call these foods what they really are: They are not "treats" for our body. They create blood sugar havoc and inflammation in our tissues. What they are is sugar-laden, dead-energy foods with no vitality. When you call it what it really is, it doesn't sound that appetizing. Visualizing the damage that sugar does to your body also helps bring you into awareness, and from a place of awareness, you are able to make a different choice.

If you choose to have the sugar-laden, dead-energy food with no vitality anyway, the second step is to ask yourself with each bite if you want to continue. See what comes up for you and try to be present with your food. Really chew thoroughly and *be* when you are eating. Give yourself permission to stop eating; it is a faulty belief that we must finish what's on our plates. Incorporating the "Seven Rs" of working with problematic thoughts and breaking the thought–emotion cycle is also useful (see Chapter 19). We need to learn to listen to the signals and messages that our body sends to indicate we are full. Ultimately, the goal is to increase our conscious, present-minded awareness and stop crossing the boundaries we have set with ourselves around eating.

Physiology

Given the basic mathematics that 3,500 calories = 1 pound, it stands to reason that either increasing your output (i.e., exercise) or decreasing your intake by 500 calories per day will result in weight loss of 1 pound per week. If this doesn't happen, you might have an underlying physiological condition (hormone imbalance) or you may not be addressing the real reason why you are eating in the first place, in the case of emotional eating.

For example, typically it takes 20 minutes for the full signal to be relayed from the nerves in your stomach to your brain. It is also interesting to note that we have approximately as many nerve endings in our entire digestive tract as we do in our spinal column. This is why it is important to learn to trust our "gut reaction," or intuition. There are more serotonin receptors in our digestive tracts than in our brains. And there is a relationship between serotonin levels and weight management. This is an important point to keep in mind, as many SSRI antidepressants have the unpleasant side effect of weight gain.

There are many hormones involved in metabolism and weight management. In addition to the hormones produced by our thyroid and adrenal glands, there are two other hormones to know about: ghrelin and leptin. If out of balance, these hormones act like gremlins and leprechauns, as they affect our ability to lose weight. Both play a role in brain chemical signalling when it comes to appetite: ghrelin is responsible for increasing hunger, and leptin is responsible for decreasing hunger. The important point is that with stress, poor eating habits and higher levels of fat, the signals from these hormones get messed up. When that happens, it is like our brain isn't listening to the signals. Just like we can become resistant to insulin, we can also become resistant to these hormones. The good news is that you can reset your brain chemistry and hormone balance to work in your favour.

Another important consideration when it comes to weight loss is the function of your organs of detoxification—in particular, the function of your liver and colon. If you find that your weight-loss efforts have reached a plateau and you are unable to lose that last 10 or 20 pounds, it can be because your organs of detoxification need attention. When we lose weight, we release stored toxins from our fat cells, and our livers have to deal with the increased demand. If your liver is not functioning optimally, it will affect your ability to lose that last 10 or 20 pounds. (See Chapter 13 for a complete discussion of your detoxification organs.) Remember that the goal of weight management is for your physiology to work with you, not against you. By ensuring optimal functioning of the organs of detoxification and assessing hormone levels, you can tip the weight-loss scales in your favour.

Exercise

REFLECTIONS FROM MY JOURNEY

I used to be of the mindset that all I needed to do was exercise more to manage my weight. To stop being bulimic, I replaced purging with increased exercise. However, this was a futile exercise based on math. If I consumed 1,000 calories while bingeing, and the extra mile I ran to compensate for what I had eaten burned 300 calories, I ended up with 700 extra calories that my body had to deal with.

If we don't immediately require the glucose that we eat, our body stores the excess as glycogen in our muscles, and when glycogen stores are full, the remaining glucose gets stored as fat. This is why it is also important to eat three meals a day and allow at least five hours between meals. If we are constantly snacking, we never give our bodies a chance to utilize our stored glycogen. When the energy demands of the body exceed what we have in our glycogen stores, the body will turn to fat as a secondary fuel source. Think of marathon runners: they are often slim because they are using all their energy sources to meet the demands of running long distances.

To manage our weight, we need to address the balance of our hormones (i.e., hypothalamic, pituitary, thyroid, adrenal and the ovarian-testes axis), change how and what we are eating, and move our bodies in ways that are fun.

I have to warn you that when you first start to eat better, you will experience the following effects: more energy, improved mood, decreased cravings, better digestion, improved concentration, increased ability to handle stress, glowing hair, skin and nails, and painless menstrual periods. Prevention is the best medicine. As Hippocrates, the father of medicine, said: "Let food be your medicine and medicine be your food."

(13)

Detoxification Organs: Colon and Liver

"Everything you put in your body informs your body."
DR. CHRIS

NOW THAT YOU have an idea of what and how to eat for optimal mental health, the next step is to make sure your digestive system and organs of elimination are supporting you as well.

Your friend, the colon

There has been much discussion lately in the media about the "gut biome" and the role bacteria play in our health, immunity and mood. It's important to understand that there is one tube from your mouth to your anus, and that tube needs to be solid, like a pipe. Near the end of the pipe (i.e., in your large colon) there are bacteria that affect not only bowel function, but also how your body handles the toxins your liver has just worked so hard at processing for elimination. Even if you've had only one round of antibiotics in your lifetime, the balance between good and bad bacteria has been disrupted. This disruption affects the terrain, or environment, in your intestines, creating a fertile ground for another opportunistic patho-gen—candida—to establish a home. You can assess whether candida is playing a role in your health by completing the questionnaire in Chapter 12.

Remember that one sign of optimal health is when you have regular, daily bowel movements. I define regular as a transit time of 12 to 18 hours. "Transit time" is the term for how long it takes you to digest, absorb and eliminate food. A simple way to determine your transit time is to eat beets. If you notice your stool has a red tinge too quickly after eating beets, it may mean that you are not getting the full benefit from your food because it is moving through your digestive tract too quickly. On the other hand, if you have a transit time greater than 18 hours, it means you are constipated, which puts your health at risk.

You can learn so much about your body by taking the time to look at your stool. Most people don't know what a healthy bowel movement should look like or how often they should have one. The result is that many people are constipated and don't even know it; or they are dependent on coffee to have a regular bowel movement—and that isn't good either because essentially you are relying on a substance (caffeine) to stimulate your bowels.

Signs of good bowel health
- Regular transit time: 12 to 18 hours.
- Shape and size: Your stool should be formed in the shape of your colon, about the length of your forearm and in an S-shape—not too hard and not too soft. It should sink to the bottom of the toilet, be uniform in colour, and be smooth, with few fissures or crevasses. There should be no blood or mucus, nor any strong, foul or offensive odour. A strong odour could indicate an imbalance in the flora or bacteria in your intestine.
- Ease: It should be easy to have a bowel movement. You shouldn't have to strain and it shouldn't hurt at all.

REFLECTIONS FROM MY JOURNEY

I had acne as a teenager and was prescribed an antibiotic (tetracycline) for several months at a time. I became constipated and would go several days without having a bowel movement. I also developed vaginal yeast infections. It is also interesting that my mental health issues started after taking these antibiotics. Research shows that there is a link between the bacteria in your digestive tract (also known as your gut biome) and your mental health. To quote a few studies:

1. There is bi-directional communication between the gut and the brain. New studies show a heavy "bottom-up" influence of the gut biome on neuronal activity in the brain. Manipulating the composition of the gut biome can have a significant impact on the brain's functioning. "Bacteria in the gastrointestinal (GI) tract can activate neural pathways and central nervous system (CNS) signaling systems."

2. Stress, a major component in many mood disorders, can alter GI flora, lowering levels of beneficial bacteria.

3. A study compared a group of patients who received a multispecies probiotic intervention with those who received a placebo. The probiotic group showed a significantly reduced incidence of ruminating thoughts—one of the most predictive habits in depressive episodes, as measured by a questionnaire indexing sensitivity (cognitive reactivity) to depression. In other words, patients become less focused on recurrent bad feelings.

I didn't make this connection between the use of antibiotics and my subsequent mental health challenges until just a few years ago. It highlights the importance of looking at one's personal history fully.

The role of the liver

The relationship between your colon and liver works like this: Your liver processes all the chemicals, toxins and hormones, and makes them water-soluble so they can be eliminated from the body. In traditional Chinese medicine, the liver is called the "master organ" because it performs many body functions, including:

- Blood purification
- Detoxification of drugs and chemicals
- Detoxification of intrinsic body toxins
- Production of enzymes and bile to help with digestion
- Hormone production
- Protein production

- Blood sugar storage and regulation
- Immune cell activation
- Storage of vitamins and iron

Due to stress, poor diet (including caffeine, sugar, trans or hydrogenated fat), alcohol, chemicals in the air, food and water, or excessive use of medications, your liver can become sluggish. The role of the liver is to take fat-soluble toxins and process them through two phases of detoxification so they can be eliminated from your body via your large colon (stool) or kidneys (urine). People do many things that end up making the first phase of detoxification go very quickly and the second phase go very slowly. It is as if there is an eight-lane highway (phase 1) waiting to merge into a one-lane highway (phase 2)—and while the cars are idling, they are spewing exhaust and polluting the environment. This is what ends up happening in your body. Toxins get broken down quickly in phase 1,and while the intermediary by-product (called a water-soluble epoxide) is waiting to be processed in phase 2, it gets recirculated via your bloodstream and contributes to inflammation. As well, there are many nutrients needed for phase 1 and 2 detoxification.

A sluggish liver results in a build-up of more toxins in your body since less detoxification is happening. An increase in toxicity leads to an increase in inflammation. If you have more inflammation from a sluggish liver, the demand for cortisol from your adrenal glands increases. Most people with anxiety and depression already suffer from a hormonal imbalance. With a cortisol imbalance, you end up suppressing neurotransmitters such as GABA, serotonin, melatonin and dopamine, all of which are related to anxiety and depression.

Also, you will require more nutrients to combat the build-up of toxins that can result in blockages around the organs. Often, it is difficult to meet the body's nutritional requirements from food alone—supplementation is required. When your liver is sluggish, it produces less bile, contributing to poor digestion. Bile is produced by the liver and stored in the gall bladder. It gets released into the small intestine when we need to process fats. It also acts as a lubricant to the large intestine as it carries toxins to be eliminated. If you don't have enough bile due to a sluggish liver, you end up constipated. With more constipation, you end up with more toxin build-up, which leads to more inflammation—and the cycle goes on. When your food is not digested properly, it creates more damage to your intestines through leaky gut syndrome.

I have a leaky what?

Think, for a moment, of the intestinal lining in your digestive tract as a tile floor. To ensure a tile floor does not leak, we put grout between the tiles. When the grout is damaged, the floor leaks. The same goes for your intestinal lining. The space between the cells (called tight junctions) is like grout, ensuring that undigested food does not make it into your body. Food must be digested all the way down to the simplest substances (glucose, minerals, vitamins, amino acids, phospholipids) to be transported across the cell wall, through the cell, back out the other side, through the space between the intestinal lining and the blood vessels, and finally into the bloodstream.

When the "grout" in the intestinal lining is damaged (due to stress, antibiotics, yeast or candida, gluten or poor diet), partially digested food can get between the cells into the area where your immune system is "on guard" waiting to attack "foreign substances." This is how we develop an IgG food intolerance known as leaky gut syndrome, or intestinal permeability. You have five immunoglobulins (Ig) at your defence: IgG, IgA, IgM, IgE and IgD. For example, an IgE immune reaction is when you have an anaphylactic or life-threatening allergic response (e.g., you eat a peanut and feel your throat closing).

With food intolerances, IgG is mounted. In an IgG reaction, the IgG antibodies attach themselves to the food antigen and create an antibody-antigen complex. These complexes are normally removed by special immune cells called macrophages. However, if they are present in large numbers and the reactive food is still being consumed, the macrophages can't keep up. The food antigen-antibody complexes accumulate and are deposited in body tissues. Once the immune system is activated, it sends inflammatory signals throughout the body that play a role in numerous diseases and conditions. This is why symptoms of food intolerances and leaky gut can appear anywhere, not just in the digestive tract.

DELAYED FOOD REACTIONS

Delayed food reactions are IgG antibody reactions (food sensitivities) that occur hours to days after you've eaten something. The inflammatory chemicals released with antibody-antigen complexes may have the following effects:

- **Systemic:** Fever, fatigue, chills, sweating and feeling weak, puffiness

- **Skin:** Itching, redness, swelling and rashes (including eczema, psoriasis)

- **Brain:** Mood and memory disturbances and behavioural problems

- **Lungs:** Bronchitis and asthma symptoms

- **Musculoskeletal:** Joint pain, muscle stiffness and swelling

- **Digestive tract:** Nausea and vomiting, diarrhea, abdominal pain, gas and bloating

Just as a drop of ink discolours an entire gallon of water, one exposure to an intolerant food can cause severe symptoms, usually within one to four days of consumption. But not only that—the exposure becomes an additional stress on the body, perpetuating the susceptibility to illness. It makes sense that the immune system reacts to the foods that are coming through—which are usually the foods you regularly eat. In treatment, the priority is to heal the leaky gut, not just to avoid the foods that are triggering the reaction.

How do you know if you have leaky gut?

There are tests available that specifically measure whether substances that don't usually traverse the intestinal lining are getting through. The most common way to identify this is by doing an IgG food intolerance test. The number and severity of IgG reactions, as well as the types of foods that show as reactive, are diagnostic for leaky gut syndrome.

CONDITIONS ASSOCIATED WITH FOOD SENSITIVITIES

Digestive disorders. Conditions like irritable bowel syndrome (IBS) and Crohn's disease have been linked to IgG food reactions. Research has shown that eliminating IgG reactive foods can alleviate IBS symptoms.

Migraines. A 2007 research study found that 43/65, or 66%, of patients with migraine headaches had complete remission of headaches after one month of eliminating reactive foods. Another study in 2010 found a significant reduction in the number of headache days and migraine attacks with elimination of reactive foods.

Mood/attention-deficit disorders. Deposition of antibody-antigen complexes in nervous system tissues may contribute to hyperactivity, depression, anxiety, inability to concentrate and other mood disorders. There is some evidence that eliminating IgG food antigens improves attentiveness in children.

Weight gain. Antibody-antigen complexes in tissue cause inflammation, which leads to fluid retention and weight gain. To fight inflammation, the body releases a chemical called ghrelin, which also happens to be an appetite stimulant. Thus, IgG food reactions may contribute to weight gain in two ways: through fluid retention and increased appetite.

How can you heal leaky gut?

The treatment we suggest at our clinic is a five-step process we call "the Five Rs":

1. Remove the offending foods.
2. Repair the GI tract.
3. Re-inoculate the digestive tract with good bacteria.
4. Restore liver function.
5. Reintroduce the foods to which you initially reacted.

Avoiding the foods that the immune system is attacking is the first step to healing leaky gut because it helps reduce inflammation and prevents further damage. Ensuring we follow the steps outlined in the previous chapters regarding diet, as well as reducing our stress levels, will further support gut healing. Also, taking digestive enzymes and probiotics helps to ensure that all food is fully digested by the time it gets to the intestines. It is also important to address intestinal yeast or candida overgrowth, heavy metal toxicity, and infections (Lyme, mono, tooth, etc.) that may be present.

The second and third step in addressing leaky gut is to take nutrients, herbs and probiotics that have been shown to heal the cells of the small intestine and support overall digestive health. These include, but are not limited to, L-glutamine,* N-acetyl glucosamine, zinc, berberine, licorice (glycyrrhizin), quercetin and aloe vera leaf extract. With probiotics, remember that there are more bacteria than there are people on the planet and it is important to introduce as many different strains of bacteria as you can. This is best achieved by rotating probiotics, as well as by eating different fermented foods (i.e., sauerkraut, kefir, kimchi, yogourt). After addressing liver function, foods can be reintroduced.

What is the impact of leaky gut?

While leaky gut syndrome is established in the naturopathic medical community, and significant research on it is coming out every year, it is not often addressed in conventional medical care. Meanwhile, it is a major underlying cause of illnesses of all sorts, in every system of the body. From chronic fatigue, sinusitis and interstitial cystitis to anxiety, depression, hypothyroidism and autoimmunity (of all types), leaky gut is both an originator and result of illness.

Stress is both a result and a cause of leaky gut, due to compromised digestion, immunity and hormone function. Supporting and rebalancing the hypothalamus-pituitary-adrenal axis is an important part of healing leaky gut.

How long does it take to heal?

Putting a stop to this snowball effect and vicious cycle associated with leaky gut is not done overnight. It requires diligence, consistency and dietary and lifestyle changes over several months or even years. The good news is that it is possible to heal. Patients report a gradual decrease in

---

* Caution is recommended with L-glutamine and bipolar disorder, as L-glutamine can increase levels of the excitatory neurotransmitter, glutamate, which can contribute to mania.

symptoms over 1 to 12 months. Overall, healing leaky gut is a key step and top priority for achieving optimal mental health.

REFLECTIONS FROM MY JOURNEY

The results of my food intolerance test identified leaky gut syndrome as I tested positive for an IgG reaction to wheat, dairy, sugar, eggs and tomatoes. Of these, I consumed wheat and sugar on a daily basis. Now, I rarely do, as I feel sluggish, bloated, irritable and anxious when I do. I didn't notice this effect before I changed my diet. What I found after eliminating these foods was that I had more energy, improved sleep, decreased mood swings, less constipation and clearer skin. A useful analogy is to view your body as a garbage can. What do you do at home when the garbage is full? You empty it. This is analogous to eliminating the foods that are a problem for you based on the test results, as these foods contribute to inflammation in the body. By taking a break, you give your detoxification organs a chance to empty the garbage. I found that when I reintroduced these foods, I had increased awareness of how these foods made me feel.

What to do if you're constipated

There are six major factors that contribute to constipation: diet, medication use, stress levels, exercise, liver function and dysbiosis (bacterial imbalances in the body). Generally, by addressing diet, stress and exercise, you will notice an improvement in bowel health. Here are a few tips to help you improve your bowel function:

1. **Avoid constipating foods** like pizza, ice cream, white bread, cheese, red meat, white flour and dairy products. Instead, follow the Mental Health Diet outlined in the Appendix. Choose leafy greens, fruit, whole grains (brown rice, millet, quinoa, etc.), beets and flaxseed oil, to name a few. And don't forget water: the minimum recommended intake is half your body weight (in pounds) in ounces of filtered or spring water every day.

2. **Optimize your digestion.** Remember what your mother always told you: Slow down and chew your food properly. Try to eat in a relaxed atmosphere and drink liquids between meals rather than with meals to support the function of your intrinsic digestive enzymes.

3. **Exercise daily.** Whether it's walking, biking, swimming, tennis, dancing, running, yoga or pilates, do an activity every day to help reduce stress and improve colon function.

4. **Don't ignore the call of nature.** If you've got to go, go. Find the nearest bathroom when you have the urge to go.

5. **Try squatting,** as it's the most natural position for elimination. Put a stool or chair in front of you to rest your feet on.

6. **Relax!** Stress is a major factor in constipation, so try to find some time to relax. If necessary, use prayer, meditation, visualization or something else that helps you relax. Take time to breathe and picture your digestive system working properly.

7. **Support your liver** by eliminating caffeine, sugar, processed foods and alcohol. By eliminating stimulants, you give the body a chance to rest and rejuvenate. Add foods that support the liver: cruciferous vegetables (broccoli, cauliflower, kale, cabbage, Brussels sprouts), bitter foods (rapini, turmeric, dandelion, nettles), grapefruit, berries, beets and fibre-containing foods.

8. **Eat organic foods as much as possible** so you don't contribute to your body's toxin load. See the Dirty Dozen and Clean Fifteen lists in Chapter 16, which outline the foods most and least sprayed with pesticides. At a minimum, pick the top three produce you are eating on the Dirty Dozen list and convert those to organic.

9. **Consult a naturopathic doctor** to get tested for digestion health (i.e., food intolerance testing for leaky gut syndrome and/or comprehensive digestive stool analysis).

10. **Consider probiotics.** If you have ever taken antibiotics, you may have an imbalance in your gut flora. Supplementation is often required, as it is difficult to get medicinal doses of healthy bacteria from food because of food manufacturing processes.

*In your **Moving Beyond** journal, make an action plan for how you will support your liver and colon based on the suggestions provided.*

Liver detoxification

If you go into a health food store, you will find many types of detoxification kits: heavy metal, liver, bowel, kidney and more. I recommend that you do detoxification or cleansing programs under the supervision of a naturopathic doctor. To assess the need to do a detoxification program, complete the Detoxification and Drainage Questionnaire on page 151. If done properly, there are five steps to a cleanse or detoxification program:

Step 1: Eat clean. Eliminate foods that slow down liver function, such as sugar, alcohol, hydrogenated fats, high-fructose corn syrup, MSG, processed foods and coffee.

Step 2: Identify causes. Complete the Environmental Quiz (in Chapter 16) to find out how to decrease the inputs that your liver must cope with.

Step 3: Support your extracellular matrix. Start homeopathic remedies to initiate the "drainage," or removal, of toxins. An extracellular matrix surrounds our tissues and organs. Imagine that I am going to deliver a letter to your front door, but there is so much clutter (quad, skis, bikes, golf clubs, hockey equipment) blocking the pathway that I can't make it to your front door, so I walk away. This is what happens to the extracellular matrix: it gets clogged with water-soluble epoxides, chemicals and heavy metals, which end up blocking receptors (the doors of the cell). Consequently, neurotransmitters, hormones, vitamins and minerals are not able to get inside the cell to do their jobs. Homeopathic drainage works on clearing the extracellular matrix so the pathway is open to the cells.

Step 4: Support liver detoxification. After the drainage process, the liver is better able to utilize nutrients. Supplements are prescribed to support phase 1 and 2 detoxification as well as the production of glutathione. Glutathione is the main anti-oxidant of the liver, which helps to get rid of toxins.

Step 5: Promote liver function. Nutrients and herbs are prescribed to promote ongoing liver function. See the list of beneficial liver foods on page 107.

In conclusion, a decrease in liver function and bile production results in poor digestion and constipation. When your food is not digested properly, your intestines can be damaged through leaky gut syndrome. This

LIVER DETOXIFICATION PATHWAYS

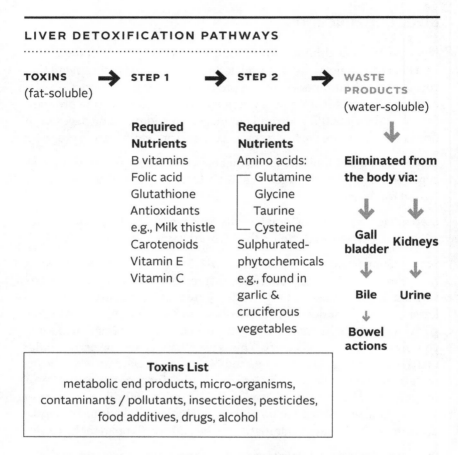

TOXINS ➡ **STEP 1** ➡ **STEP 2** ➡ WASTE
(fat-soluble)   PRODUCTS
                                                  (water-soluble)

Required   **Required**   ⬇
Nutrients   **Nutrients**
B vitamins   Amino acids: **Eliminated from**
Folic acid   ┌ Glutamine   **the body via:**
Glutathione   │ Glycine
Antioxidants   │ Taurine   ⬇   ⬇
e.g., Milk thistle   └ Cysteine
Carotenoids   Sulphurated-   **Gall**   **Kidneys**
Vitamin E   phytochemicals   **bladder**
Vitamin C   e.g., found in
                      garlic &   ⬇   ⬇
                      cruciferous
                      vegetables   **Bile**   **Urine**

                                                   ⬇
                                                   Bowel
                                                   actions

Toxins List
metabolic end products, micro-organisms,
contaminants / pollutants, insecticides, pesticides,
food additives, drugs, alcohol

is when you have gaps in your intestinal lining that allow more toxins to enter your bloodstream and create more inflammation in your body. When you have a sluggish liver, you have poor digestion, which means you have fewer nutrients available to create neurotransmitters.

Basically, to recap, a sluggish liver contributes to poor digestion, which leads to reduced brain function, which can be a root cause of mood disturbances.

DO YOU NEED A DETOX?
....

Try the following Detoxification and Drainage Questionnaire to determine whether symptoms you're experiencing could be related to a need for detoxification.

POINT COUNT	POINTS
Never or almost never have the symptom	0
Occasionally have it, effect is not severe	1
Occasionally have it, effect is severe	2
Frequently have it, effect is not severe	3
Frequently have it, effect is severe	4

EMOTIONS

Irritability _____

Nervousness _____

Mood swings _____

Frequent crying _____

Aggressive behaviour, i.e., road rage _____

Anxiety _____

Fear _____

Confusion _____

Depression _____

Suicidal thoughts _____

TOTAL EMOTIONS SCORE _____

SKIN

Increased sweating, ear wax, oily skin _____

Skin rashes _____

Brown spots on hands and face _____

Boils _____

Skin tags (small hanging warts) _____

Acne _____

Eczema _____

Fever blisters   _____
Warts   _____

TOTAL SKIN SCORE   _____

EAR, NOSE AND THROAT
Increased salivation   _____
Mouth ulcers   _____
Common cold   _____
Sinusitis   _____
Sore throat   _____
Ear infections   _____
Hay fever   _____
Loss of smell   _____
Cough   _____

TOTAL EAR, NOSE AND THROAT SCORE   _____

MIND AND BRAIN
Hyperactivity   _____
Stammering when speaking
    or problem finding words   _____
Difficulty in concentration   _____
Difficulty in making decisions   _____
Headache   _____
Poor memory   _____
Poor coordination   _____
Compulsive behaviour   _____
Sleep disturbance   _____
Memory loss   _____

TOTAL MIND AND BRAIN SCORE   _____

DIGESTIVE SYSTEM

Loose stools   _____

Diarrhea   _____

Heartburn   _____

Constipation   _____

Bloating   _____

Abdominal pain   _____

Intolerance to certain foods   _____

Nausea or vomiting   _____

Severe diarrhea with blood or mucus   _____

TOTAL DIGESTIVE SYSTEM SCORE   _____

KIDNEY

Increase in urination frequency and amount   _____

Kidney stones   _____

Blood in the urine   _____

Needing to get up in the night to pass urine   _____

Urinary tract infections and cystitis   _____

TOTAL KIDNEY SCORE   _____

JOINTS AND MUSCLES

Muscle aches or joint aches   _____

Tendinitis (e.g., tennis elbow, golfer's
   elbow, Achilles tendinitis)   _____

Gout   _____

Arthritis   _____

Fibromyalgia   _____

TOTAL JOINTS AND MUSCLE SCORE   _____

METABOLISM

Feeling of coldness	_____
Hypoglycemia	_____
Craving certain foods	_____
Water retention	_____
Obesity	_____
Cellulite	_____

TOTAL METABOLISM SCORE _____

GRAND TOTAL SCORE _____

SCORE:

High toxic load: > 50* ~ A supervised detoxification program is highly recommended.

Moderate: 15–49 ~ A supervised detoxification program is recommended.

Low: < 14 ~ A detoxification program is not needed.

* With scores greater than 50, other mechanisms should be considered, such as inflammation/immune/allergic gastrointestinal function, oxidative stress, hormonal/neurotransmitter dysfunction, nutritional depletion and/or mind-body imbalances. Individualized support with specific medical foods, diet and/or nutraceuticals prescribed by a naturopathic doctor is recommended.

(14)

Sleep

"There is no quick-fix solution to multifactorial conditions."
DR. CHRIS

SLEEP IS ESSENTIAL to everyone. It is a time when your brain and body balance and regulate their vital systems to prepare for the next day. A lack of sleep deprives your brain and body of this essential rest period and can compromise your ability to get through the day successfully. Can you think back to a time when you were sleep deprived? What happened? Did you get sick? Did you lose your patience more easily? Did you use stimulants to get through the day?

There can be a few issues when it comes to sleep. It is important to work with a naturopathic doctor to get to the root cause or causes of your sleep concerns. Indications that you are not getting enough sleep are:

- Sleeping in
- Hitting the snooze button repeatedly
- Not feeling rested in the morning
- Needing to use caffeine to "wake up"
- Needing to nap during the day
- Mood instability
- Decreased productivity at work
- Weight gain
- Low libido
- Impaired judgment

⚬⚊➤ *Write in your **Moving Beyond** journal about how you feel if you don't get enough sleep. What are your thoughts on sleep? Do you have a sleep routine? Do you have any of the above indications that you aren't getting enough sleep?*

Sleep is often overlooked in the pursuit of optimal health. Insomnia, and its resultant effect on mood, is one of the most common health concerns I see in practice. With the explosion of technology, social media, Wi-Fi, the Internet and all our devices, we are compromising our long-term health with our short-term fixation on the latest status update, tweet, Instagram post or YouTube video.

The quality of your sleep, not only the number of hours you get, is important. After I had my son, I found myself joking that I didn't think my sleep would return to normal until he moved out of the house. But all kidding aside, it is important to do what you can to get the sleep you need. (This is often difficult when you have a newborn or young children—you may have to endure less than optimal sleep at this time!)

REFLECTIONS FROM MY JOURNEY

Since I have had many challenges in the sleep department—from not being able to fall sleep, to disrupted sleep, to being unable to fall back to sleep, to sleeping all day long—I hope that you can learn from me in how I manage my sleep. I treat sleep like a precious commodity and feel that regardless of your health affliction, sleep is a critical component to getting well.

If you're not waking up feeling rested, there are a few possible patterns to investigate:

· Difficulty falling asleep
· Difficulty staying asleep
· Difficulty falling *and* staying asleep
· Insufficient sleep (staying up too late or waking up too early)
· Insufficient sleep that is also interrupted

Depending on what category you fall into, your mood may be affected.

Difficulty falling asleep

A common issue with sleep is difficulty falling asleep. To address this, I typically start with lifestyle suggestions around sleep (see page 164) and encourage journalling, eliminating caffeine and eliminating sugar. If you can't eliminate these entirely, then don't have caffeine after 12 p.m. or sugar after 6 p.m. Many people use alcohol to fall asleep, but this is a slippery slope: the half-life of wine, for example, is four hours. Its effects start to wear off at that point, causing some people to wake up.

Many people are on their phones or devices before bed. This is also a big problem because of the blue light and electromagnetic energy they emit. It is important to unplug from our TVs, phones and computers at least one hour before bed. I personally try to avoid using the computer or checking my phone two hours before bed. This is because I don't want to be triggered by a negative news event prior to going to sleep. It is best to do what you can to protect yourself from any negativity or upsetting discussions before bed. I take this very seriously and do my best to avoid the news like the plague. The last thing I want to see before I go to sleep is something negative. Sleep is a precious commodity and needs to be valued and protected as such.

Difficulty staying asleep

Sleep is also important to the rhythm of our adrenal glands, which produce many hormones, including cortisol. Ideally, we would go to bed and get up at the same time each day. Cortisol has a diurnal rhythm in the body, which means it is naturally high in the morning and low at night. It can also inhibit the sleep hormone, melatonin, since it has an inverse relationship with melatonin.

If you are staying up late playing video games online or scrolling through your social media accounts, the increased stimulation can result in a rise in cortisol at the exact time when your body is trying to produce melatonin. It may be difficult to fall asleep, and sleep may escape you because you are producing too much cortisol, inhibiting melatonin production.

For the person who has no problem falling asleep but wakes up at 3 a.m. to go to the bathroom and can't get back to sleep because their

HOW HORMONES AFFECT YOUR SLEEP:
The Relationship Between Cortisol and Melatonin

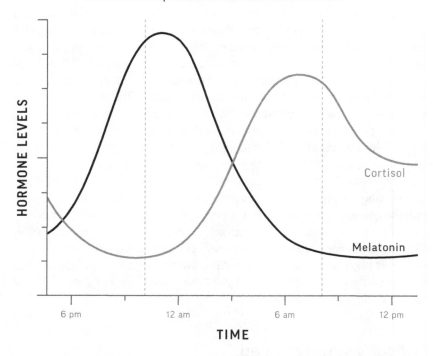

It's ideal to wake up with a full tank of gas in the morning. This means optimal levels of cortisol. More often in practice, I see the opposite cortisol curve in patients: low levels in the morning and high levels at night.

mind is suddenly switched on by thinking about work, this can also cause cortisol to rise, inhibiting melatonin and making it difficult to fall back asleep. In practice, I find there are two ways to deal with this problem. Remember the tryptophan pathway chart on page 95. The first step in the formation of melatonin is the conversion of tryptophan to 5-hydroxytryptophan (5-HTP). When taken at bedtime, 5-HTP metabolizes into melatonin over the course of the night, giving a boost to melatonin levels that may be dropping in someone who has an early rising cortisol rhythm. The other strategy is to prescribe herbs and nutrients to calm cortisol, such as magnolia bark or phosphatidylserine.

It's ideal to wake up with a full tank of gas in the morning. This means optimal levels of cortisol. More often in practice, I see the opposite cortisol curve in patients: low levels in the morning and high levels at night.

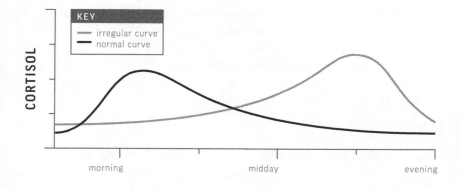

The dark line in the cortisol curve diagram is showing a healthy cortisol curve; the light line is not. In addition to cortisol, estrogen and progesterone also pay a role in sleep; their levels may need to be investigated as well. It is common practice among naturopathic doctors to measure hormone levels to see if these are playing a role in sleep.

You can determine the health of your adrenal glands by completing the following Adrenal Stress Indicator test. Depending on your symptoms, further testing may be required to assess the functioning of your adrenal glands. Naturopathic doctors often recommend a salivary cortisol curve test to determine the diurnal rhythm of cortisol production.

ADRENAL STRESS INDICATORS

Write the number 1 beside symptoms you have had in the past; 2 beside symptoms that occur occasionally; 3 beside symptoms that occur often; and 4 beside symptoms that occur frequently.

Add up the score.

_____ Blurred vision/spots in front of eyes

_____ Hormonal imbalances (i.e. thyroid problems)

_____ History of asthma/bronchitis

_____ Prolonged exposure to stress (job, family, illness, caregiving)

_____ Headaches

_____ Environmental or chemical exposure or sensitivities

_____ Hypoglycemia/blood sugar problems-mood swings

_____ Food allergies

_____ Poor concentration/memory problems (Alzheimer's disease)

_____ Low energy, excessive fatigue

_____ Easily overwhelmed, inability to handle stress

_____ Post-exertion fatigue

_____ Dizziness upon standing (or fainting)

_____ Inflammatory conditions (arthritis, bursitis)

_____ Nervousness/anxiety, depression, irritability or anger

_____ Shortness of breath/yawning (air hunger)

_____ Cold hands or feet

_____ Low back pain, knee problems, sore muscles

_____ Insomnia/frequent waking

_____ Excessive urination

_____ Excessive perspiration or no perspiration

_____ Heart palpitations

_____ Edema of extremities or general edema

_____ Eyes light-sensitive

_____ Cravings: sugar, salt, coffee or other stimulants

_____ Alcohol intolerance

_____ Recurrent cold or infections

_____ Digestive problems, ulcers

_____ Weight gain or weight loss

_____ High or low blood pressure

_____ **TOTAL SCORE**

INTERPRETING YOUR SCORE

If you scored...

- **BETWEEN 30 AND 50:** you've received an early-warning indicator that your adrenals are starting to weaken.

- **BETWEEN 50 AND 80:** Start with an adrenal support as recommended by your naturopathic doctor.

- **BETWEEN 80 AND 100:** Your adrenals are taxed. You may want to take an adrenal glandular product as recommended by your naturopathic doctor.

- **OVER 100:** You are suffering from adrenal exhaustion and will require long-term adrenal support. Please schedule an appointment with a naturopathic doctor.

Reproduced with permission from *The Adrenal Stress Connection* by Dr. Karen Jensen, ND, and Dr. Marita Schauch, BSC, ND.

Waking up

So much of the discussion around mental health and sleep is about getting to sleep, but I would be remiss if I didn't discuss how to get out of bed in the morning. When I am depressed, I can sleep forever! I am often amazed at how much I can sleep: 16 to 18 hours per day for days on end. Just as a decrease in sleep is a reason to seek medical attention, the reverse is also true. If you have one or two days where you don't get out of bed, this can be one of the first signs that you are slipping into a depressive episode.

At one point, I was prescribed Dexedrine, an amphetamine used in attention-deficit hyperactivity disorder (ADHD), to help keep me awake during the day. I found that this led me to be more anxious, and I didn't like the idea of taking a stimulant that has a high potential for addiction.

From a naturopathic perspective, it is often the hypothalamus-pituitary-adrenal (HPA) axis that needs nurturing when someone is not able to get out of bed. It is also important to look at why you can't get out of bed. Is it due to your physical energy? Is it because you don't want to face the day? Is it because you are suicidal? Is it all of the above? It is important to determine what the root issue is and then take steps to correct the situation. Mental health conditions, such as depression, anxiety and bipolar disorder, often require a helping hand from a spouse, family member, caregiver or close friend. I know for me it has been extremely hard to reach out and ask for help when I am in a deep depression. Asking a depressed person to reach out for help is like asking a blind person to see or a deaf person to hear: we are physically challenged in that area. This is why it is important to discuss coping and implementation strategies with your loved ones when you are well. That way, if you slip into a depression, you won't have to ask for help; they will know what to do to help you. One of the strategies that is important to put in place, especially if you are prone to sleeping the day away, is to meet someone for a walk by 10 a.m. in the morning.

O— *How you live your day is how you start your day. In your* **Moving Beyond** *journal, write about ways your support group can help you get out of bed in the morning. Ideas are: play an uplifting song, take you for a walk, feed you breakfast, bring you water.*

Mania discussion

In terms of preventing mania, I think sleep and stress management are critical. I advise my patients to get in touch with me if they have a sleepless night, as I want to help them prevent a manic episode. Personally, if I had a sleepless night, I would be fearful that this was an indication I was heading into a manic episode. I have since learned that worrying does not support my health in a positive way because all it does is turn on the stress response, which is counterproductive to supporting sleep. As mentioned earlier, the stress hormone (cortisol) inhibits our ability to produce the sleep hormone (melatonin). For women, if you notice that your sleep quality is disrupted prior to menstruation, this can indicate low progesterone levels. Please see a naturopathic doctor, who can determine if this is a factor in your case. I find this is important to consider at the time of perimenopause/menopause.

REFLECTIONS FROM MY JOURNEY

As someone with bipolar disorder type 1, I can tell you that sleep is a critical foundation of my mental health. I have worked very hard to move from the place of fear around my sleep (for example, worry I might go manic if I have a suboptimal night of sleep) to a place where I am at peace with the sleep I get and learning to trust the wisdom of my body to get the sleep I need. An important rule that I have adopted is that if I have two consecutive nights of suboptimal sleep, I will call either my naturopathic doctor or my psychiatrist for support. I encourage you to do the same. Sleep, and managing the stress associated with it, is the best ways to prevent mania from occurring.

Everyone has different needs when it comes to sleep. Whatever your ideal number of hours is, I would urge you to protect it the same way you would protect anything else that is precious to you: it is *that* important. And depending on what mental health condition you are trying to resolve, protecting it may be critical—as in the case of bipolar disorder. On the flip side, if you are depressed and tend to sleep all day, or have no desire to get out of bed, that needs to be addressed too.

Getting a better sleep

Here are some lifestyle suggestions to support your sleep. I encourage you to check off what you are already doing and incorporate as many suggestions as you can to support healthy sleep hygiene.

1. Stimulants

- **Avoid or minimize things that could be too stimulating** two hours before bed. This includes violent TV shows or movies, news, computer games, smart phones, social media, arguments and important discussions. These are too stimulating to the brain. They disrupt your pineal gland function and will cause you to take longer to fall asleep.

- **Avoid alcohol** (wine, beer and hard liquor) two hours before bed. The effect of alcohol is short-lived. People will often wake up several hours later, unable to fall back to sleep. Alcohol will also keep you from falling into the deeper stages of sleep, where the body does most of its healing.

- **Avoid food, beverages and medications containing caffeine** (such as pop, tea, coffee, chocolate, coffee-flavoured ice cream and diet pills) after 12 noon. Better yet, try to quit caffeine all together by slowly tapering down over time. Caffeine contributes to the need to urinate frequently, which is disruptive to sleep.

- **Avoid drinking more than an 8-ounce cup of fluids** before going to bed.

- **Avoid decongestant cold medicines** at night, and ask your pharmacist or doctor whether any other medications you regularly take may have stimulating effects. (But do not discontinue them without permission from your doctor.)

- **Avoid large meals** close to bedtime. Large meals may lead to reflux, heartburn and other digestive concerns, which may result in poor sleep.

- **Avoid exercise** close to bedtime; do it at least three hours before bedtime.

- **Avoid cigarettes.** Cigarettes are a stimulant and make it difficult to fall asleep. Also, because their chemical effects wear off quickly, your sleep will be disrupted due to withdrawal. You may notice this by needing to have a cigarette immediately on waking.

- **Lose weight.** Being overweight can increase the risk of sleep apnea, which will prevent a restful night's sleep.

2. Evening tension and anxiety

- **Avoid paying bills** before bed. Avoid checking your banking accounts, financial reports or stock market results.

- **Schedule difficult conversations** at least three hours before going to sleep. Try to reach a resolution before bed.

- **Do NOT watch the clock.** Better yet, remove the clock from your view. Constantly staring at it will cause more worry.

- **Try the Emotional Freedom Technique.** This can be a wonderful sleep aid. Most people can learn this simple and gentle tapping technique in several minutes. It can help balance your body's bioenergetic system and resolve some of the emotional stresses that are contributing to insomnia on a very deep level. The results are typically long-lasting and the improvement is remarkably rapid.

- **Sleep in a separate room** if your partner snores loudly or tosses and turns and you find your sleep is being interrupted. Do this if you need to. There is nothing wrong with it.

- **Try guided imagery or progressive/systematic** relaxation if you are not asleep within 30 minutes of going to bed.

3. Thoughts and common worries about sleep

- **Use positive self-talk.** Repeat or write out a positive affirmation in your journal regarding sleep. I encourage you to write it out 10 times in a row and do this three times a day. Here is one I use: "I trust in the wisdom of my body to get the sleep I need."

- **Avoid excessive worrying** about insomnia, as it may be more detrimental to your health than the sleep loss itself. The most likely consequence of not getting enough sleep is that you will feel tired and irritable. Although these are uncomfortable inconveniences, they are not catastrophic. Shift from worry to trust.

- **Avoid negative judgments** about the fact that you are unable to sleep.

- **Keep a sleep diary** to help you be more realistic and affirm that you experience a good night's sleep more often than you may realize.

- **Write down and challenge negative thoughts.** Regardless of how your insomnia started, how you think and behave can contribute to prolonging it. As you control your thoughts, you can improve your sleep patterns. It may be beneficial to see a cognitive behavioural therapist for additional support.

- **Don't panic about a poor night's sleep.** This makes your sleep worse. Trust in your body's wisdom that you are getting enough sleep.

- **Instead of trying to fall asleep, do the opposite** and try to stay awake. Taking away the pressure of "needing" to sleep could help you fall asleep.

- **Manage your expectations** and be patient. Your disturbed sleep patterns have taken time to learn, and it may take a while to unlearn them.

4. Sleep planning and bedroom preparation

- **Reserve your bed for sleeping.** If you watch TV or work in bed, you may find it harder to relax and to think of the bed as a place to sleep.

- **Plan** to get to get seven to nine hours of sleep per night.

- **Only go to bed when you are sleepy.** Lying in bed trying to sleep when you're not tired will increase your frustration.

- **Have a bedtime ritual.** Brushing your teeth, having a relaxing bath, washing your face, getting your pyjamas on, or reading, for example, help to signal the body and brain that it is time to sleep.

- **Take a warm bath, shower or sauna one or two hours before bed.** When your body temperature rises late in the evening, it will fall at bedtime, facilitating sleep.

- **Keep a regular routine and avoid getting to bed after midnight.** Get to bed as early as possible and at the same time each night. Following a regular routine helps train our biological clocks. The body needs to know when it is supposed to sleep. Our body recharges during the hours of 11p.m. to 1 a.m. In addition, your gallbladder dumps toxins during this period. If you are awake, the toxins back up into the liver, which backs up into your entire system and causes further disruption to your health.

- **Avoid late afternoon or evening naps,** as these can disrupt your night-time sleep.

- **Consider reading** something spiritual before bed to encourage relaxation. Don't read anything stimulating, such as a mystery or suspense novel, as this may have the opposite effect. If you are really enjoying a suspenseful book, you may wind up unintentionally reading for hours instead of going to sleep. Other positive wind-down activities include listening to relaxing music or following a guided meditation.

- **Do journalling.** If you often lie in bed with your mind racing, or wake up and can't go back to sleep because of your thoughts, it might be helpful to keep a journal and write your thoughts down before bed. Personally, I have been doing this for many years, and I find it helps tremendously. You can also write your thoughts out in the morning to help start your day on the right foot. I love journalling so much that I published *Moving Beyond: A Journal into Self-Discovery*.

   If you have trouble falling asleep or wake up in the middle of the night and can't return to sleep, **don't lie in bed for more than 45 minutes** trying to fall asleep. Utilize sleep techniques, such as reading with low light, word puzzles, Sudoku, knitting, progressive relaxation, journalling or meditation.

- **Do alternate nostril breathing** 10 minutes before bed, which helps to restore the circadian rhythm and increases the amount of melatonin produced by the body at night.

5. Foods

- **Eat a light, tryptophan-forming snack** an hour before bed. High-protein snacks like turkey, fish, poultry and eggs are best. (See the Appendix section "Eating for Mental Wellness," for more foods that are high in tryptophan.)

- **Avoid foods that you may be sensitive to.** This is particularly true for dairy and wheat products, as they may influence sleep. In some people, they can cause sleep apnea, excess congestion, gastrointestinal upset, gas and other symptoms.

- **Avoid sugars, carbohydrates and grains one to two hours before bed.** This includes chocolate, cookies, sweets, bread, cereal, crackers and so on. Such foods will raise your blood sugar levels and inhibit sleep. Later, when blood sugar levels drop too low (hypoglycemia), you might wake up and not be able to fall back to sleep.

6. Bedroom air quality and environment

- **Use an air purifier or filter** (one with HEPA, or high-efficiency particulate arrestance, is best) to clean the air in your bedroom. Use the filter on a low setting if the noise is soothing. Otherwise, use the filter on a medium setting for four to six hours during the day.

- **Clean the vents** in your house once a year and change your furnace filters every three months if you have forced-air heating.

- **Reduce nasal congestion** by dusting your room. Consider using a saline spray, breathe-easy strips or warming socks hydrotherapy.

- **Dress comfortably** for bed.

- **Wear socks to bed.** Feet have poor circulation and as a result, they often feel cold before the rest of the body does. At least one study has shown that wearing socks to bed reduces night waking.

- **Ensure the temperature** in your bedroom is neither too hot nor too cold.

- **Check your bedroom for electromagnetic fields (EMF),** which disrupt the pineal gland and the production of melatonin. You can use a gauss meter to measure EMFs. Dr. Herbert Ross, author of *Sleep Disorders*, even recommends people pull their circuit breaker before bed to kill all power in the house.

- **Remove smart phones and fitness trackers from your bedroom** because these are EMF producers. The irony, of course, is that fitness trackers are designed to measure your sleep quality—but in the process of doing so, they emit EMFs. Many in the field of environmental medicine feel that using a fitness tracker is counterproductive and may be a contributing factor in disrupting your sleep. Our society has become too dependent on gadgets. Do you really need a fitness tracker to tell you your sleep is off?

- **Keep your head at least five feet away from electric fields.** Possible sources of electrical fields include electrical outlets, clock radios, stereos, smart phones, fitness trackers, computers and monitors. While this is recommended, my bedroom has never been big enough to accommodate this and it is too cold where I live for most of the year to sleep outside in a tent away from all electrical outlets. While the electrical outlet is near my bed, I only have a lamp plugged into it, and I have a battery-operated clock on my nightstand that doesn't emit any light.

- **Avoid water beds or electric blankets** because of excessive heat and EMFs.

7. Light and noise

- **Turn down the light** in the bathroom and any other rooms you are in 15 minutes before going to bed. Decrease the light in your bedroom by using a dimmer or a lower-watt bulb in the lamp beside your bed.

- **Sleep in complete darkness** or as close to it as possible. Consider using black-out blinds or eye shades. This prevents early waking due to sunlight. When light hits the eyes, it disrupts the circadian rhythm of the pineal gland and the production of melatonin. There should also be as little light in the bathroom as possible if you get up in the middle of the night.

- **Eliminate loud noises** with earplugs (recommend: Ohropax brand) or add white noise, such as a fan or soft music. Ensure windows are closed, and turn off or remove any appliances or clocks that make noise.

- **Use an alarm clock without lights** that has a gentle alarm. It is stressful on the body to be woken up suddenly with an obnoxious alarm or to blaring music. If you are getting enough sleep, alarm clocks are not necessary. Consider the use of a dawn simulator, which turns the light on gradually, reaching full intensity after 45 minutes.

8. Bedding and pillows

- **Consider replacing your pillows** with ultrafine hypoallergenic pillows if you have a dust allergy.

- **Wash your pillows** at least twice a year.

- **Use a body pillow** to hug and put between your knees to align your back and shoulders at night. Roll backwards at a slight angle onto a body pillow if you have hip bursitis.

- **Use lavender.** Sprinkle clean sheets and pillowcases with lavender water. The scent is proven to promote relaxation. Lavender essential oil in a diffuser can promote a calm environment in your bedroom.

9. Supplements and medications

- **Take mineral supplements** at bedtime (magnesium and/or calcium).

- **Discuss natural sleep aids** with a naturopathic doctor.

- **Reduce or avoid as many medications as possible.** Many medications, both prescription and over-the-counter, may have a negative effect on sleep.

- **Have your hormones checked by a naturopathic doctor.** Scientists have found that insomnia may be caused by hormone imbalances. This can affect men as well as women. Depending on your hormonal stage of life—for example, menopause or perimenopause in women or andropause in men—sleep quality can be affected.

REFLECTIONS FROM MY JOURNEY

We cannot underestimate the relationship between having a healthy sleep routine and having a balanced mood. I used to hit the snooze button five or even ten times before I could drag myself out of bed. Then I would be in a frenetic rush to get to work on time. I never thought I would see the day where I would wake up at 6 a.m. after eight hours of sleep feeling rested and full of energy. So, you can imagine my shock and delight when this actually happened to me. This is a sign of healthy adrenal function, something we all can achieve.

Here is my sleep routine:

1. Get to bed by 9:30 or 10 p.m.
2. Ensure there is no light stimulation from electronics after 8 p.m. and no TV after 10 p.m.

3. Journal until my mind feels empty, calm and at peace, as I have let go of whatever is weighing on me.
4. Meditate for 10 to 30 minutes.
5. At the end of journalling and meditation, I ask myself the following question: Do I need to take anything to help me sleep (whether natural or pharmaceutical)? And I trust the answer that comes from my intuition.
6. If the answer is yes, I take natural sleeps aids as prescribed by my naturopathic doctor (magnesium bisglycinate, melatonin, 5-HTP, botanical medicines and/or homeopathic remedies).
7. Read until I fall asleep. I typically read anywhere from 5 to 30 minutes before I turn the light off and fall asleep.
8. If I don't fall asleep immediately, I will pray. If my thoughts interrupt me, I will keep restarting at the beginning of the prayer.
9. If sleep doesn't come by 1 a.m., I may repeat Steps 1 to 8 until I fall asleep. Depending on what I have going on the next day, I may resort to a pharmaceutical medication, such as lorazepam (Ativan). However, this is extremely rare and typically happens fewer than three times a year. I am mindful of my thoughts, and do not go to the place of fear in my mind. This has taken me a long time to understand, given my experience with mania. I feel that sleep has been a critical component in maintaining my mental well-being.
10. Get out of bed after being in bed for a maximum of 10 hours.

I want you to know that I've been stuck in depression for years, and during that time, I slept much of my life away. I know that depression steals you away from your life, and I know that you may need extra sleep when you are depressed. I encourage you to develop structure and a routine and to enlist support if needed.

As discussed at the outset of this chapter, poor sleep can have a variety of root causes, so it is important to work with a naturopathic doctor to get to the heart of your sleep concerns. Since I have had many challenges in the sleep department—from not being able to fall sleep, to disrupted sleep, to being unable to fall back asleep, to sleeping all day long—I hope you can learn from me in. I treat sleep like a precious commodity and feel that regardless of your health affliction, it is a critical component to maintaining wellness.

Ultimately, your day needs to start on the right foot. To "wake up on the right side of the bed," you need to get adequate sleep. Being productive and getting the most out of your waking hours starts with sleeping well at night. We need to support our sleep, not sacrifice it. How we feel throughout the day—tired, exhausted and depleted or vibrant, enthusiastic and energized—is profoundly affected by our sleep patterns.

There are many different theories about what is best, and what might be right for one person may not be the same for another, given differences in stress, work obligations, number of children, and many other factors. My recommendation is that you aim for seven to nine hours of sleep per night. Most people are sleep deprived. If they could improve their sleep, perhaps they would have more energy, patience and productivity, better time management, and less road rage and other stress. Ultimately, you are the only person who knows how you feel in your body and how much sleep is best for you.

(15)

Exercise

"I have never once come back from exercising outside
feeling worse than when I started."
DR. CHRIS

THE MOOD DISORDERS Society of Canada published a startling statistic in 2009: one in five Canadians will experience a mental illness
in their lifetime, whether depression, anxiety disorder, bipolar disorder, schizophrenia, ADHD or dementia (with anxiety and depression
being the most common by far). If 20% of our population will experience
such an event, it is very likely you or someone you know is, has been
or will be affected by mental illness. Rates have been climbing steadily
in Canada for several decades and are expected to continue increasing.
Within a generation, it is estimated that more than 8.9 million Canadians
will be living with a mental illness.

Nearly 10% of our country's population is using some form of prescription antidepressant medication. The economic burden of mental
illness in Canada is estimated at $51 billion per year. This includes health
care costs, lost productivity, and reductions in health-related quality of
life. With so many Canadians living with mental illness, together with
such high treatment costs, it's a wonder that one of the most effective,
safe and inexpensive tools for mood regulation is so underused as a pre-
scriptive treatment for mental illness: exercise.

When I lecture and speak to patients, I share a popular health and wellness assertion that pharmaceuticals (antidepressants) are the most over-utilized prescription for depression and anxiety and that exercise is the most under-utilized. I go on to explain that I understand how difficult it is when you are in the pit of depression and despair to exercise. I also share that there have been times when that is all that I have "accomplished" in a day. The struggle to get myself out the door has been agony at times. It has taken me several hours—two, four, six, eight or 10 hours at times—to move from my bedroom to the back door. When I am depressed, the battle between the side of me that wants to get well and the side of me that is stuck in depression and defeat can be paralyzing, and it can take hours to muster up the courage to do all the steps required to get outside:

1. Get out of bed.
2. Get dressed.
3. Brush my teeth or hair if I am not able to take a shower.
4. Get to the door.
5. Put my shoes on.
6. Open the door.
7. Take one step.
8. Take another step.
9. Take another step.
10. Repeat Steps 8 and 9 for a minimum of 30 minutes.

REFLECTIONS FROM MY JOURNEY

Sometimes I have sat at the door for over an hour just struggling with the contemplation and action of putting my shoes on. But, I can tell you this, as much as I didn't want to go, I have never once come back from exercising outside feeling worse than when I began. Never. Once. The endorphin benefit may be short-lived and may not sustain me to the next morning, but I believe that there is a cumulative effect of exercise and that if you repeat it enough times on a weekly or daily basis, you can't help but feel better. I know it seems hard. But I also know that you will feel better. Exercise can be addictive because of the endorphin release that affects our brain chemistry. Just like food, it needs to be monitored, especially if you have an eating disorder. It is important to work with all-or-nothing beliefs (since all-or-nothing thinking is a thinking style strongly linked with depression) to find the balance point that supports your health.

It seems almost too easy to think that something as simple as exercise could have a real impact on mental illness, but strong evidence speaks loudly. Studies on the neurobiochemistry of mental illness show exercise is an effective treatment.

What kind of exercise?

Aerobic, resistance and strength training, recreational, and "green exercise"
Many studies investigating the beneficial effects of exercise on mental health are done on aerobic exercise, generally 60 to 300 minutes per week of aerobic activity: jogging, cycling and other such high-intensity activities. Research reviews on aerobic exercise show significant reductions in depression and anxiety scores, improved cognition, and improved self-perception—features central to many mental health improvements. A 2016 meta-analysis focusing on regular aerobic exercise as a treatment for depression shows it is statistically equal to antidepressants as treatment, without any of the cost or adverse effects. When exercise is used in combination with medication, response is better than either treatment alone. Several studies have also shown aerobic exercise to be effective at reducing psychiatric symptoms in individuals diagnosed with schizophrenia, bipolar disorder, ADHD or obsessive-compulsive disorder.

Fortunately, it's not just running and aerobics that improve mental health. Studies have also shown the psychological benefit of regular strength and resistance training without aerobic fitness improvement. Regular weight lifting, playing sports and other types of active exercise can improve mood and decrease anxiety and depression scores just as well as rigorous, high-intensity running can. These improvements to mental well-being can begin to be seen with as little as 20 minutes three to five times a week of brisk walking, tennis, dancing, weight training or anything else that gets your heart rate up or your muscles pumping.

A review of population-wide studies in the United States and Canada tells another interesting story about what type of exercise is best for the brain—it's more beneficial when it's recreational. Compiling data and comparing groups of people who use similar amounts of energy in household chores versus recreational exercise shows a greater psychological benefit among the group engaging in recreational exercise.

Finally, to get the most out of exercise, take it outside. It is known that both physical activity and exposure to nature separately have positive effects on physical and mental health. Research is now showing they have a synergistic effect on parameters of mental health when experienced together. Their combination is being called "green exercise," and it is proven to be more beneficial than exercise without exposure to nature. A 2010 study shows that the perceived greenness of an exercise area (meaning how natural the environment is) is proportionally correlated with reductions in anxiety after exercising there. In other words, the greener the environment of your walk or run, the less anxious you will feel after you've done it. Another study reports significantly improved blood pressure, mood and self-esteem after running in pleasant natural environments versus control environments like running on a treadmill without a screen or in unpleasant environments. A meta-analysis shows that the people affected most positively by the presence of nature during exercise are those suffering from mental health concerns.

Who benefits from exercise?

The significant, measurable psychological effects described above are seen in both clinical populations (those with a diagnosed anxious or depressive disorder) and in healthy populations, which highlights the fact that exercise benefits both those with mental illness and those wanting to prevent it. This effect is seen in all ages, from adolescents to the elderly. It is interesting to note that the positive effect of exercise on parameters of mental health is independent of economic status, age, gender and physical health status. This means a person can start wherever they are—fit or not, young or old—and still feel the psychological benefits of exercise.

How exercise supports mental health

Various mechanisms are responsible for the mental health benefits of exercise. The first and perhaps most obvious physiological changes that happen during exercise are increased heart and breathing rates. This allows for higher oxygen delivery to the whole body, including the brain. Increased cerebral vascular flow sends nutrients, energy and other benefits to brain cells to support their function during the strain of physical exertion. It even changes the patterns of neuronal activity post-exercise. For example, changing blood flow and brain metabolism through exercise has been shown to alter symptomatic neural response in adults and children with bipolar disorder. Several studies are proposing physical activity as a new early treatment of this condition.

Increased blood flow to the brain activates the metabolic pathways that replenish depleted neurotransmitters, a circumstance common to many mental health disorders. Dr. Richard Maddock, a professor in the Department of Psychiatry and Behavioral Sciences at the University of California Davis, explains, "From a metabolic standpoint, vigorous exercise is the most energetically demanding activity the brain encounters, much more intense than calculus or chess, and one of the things it's doing [with all the energy] is making more neurotransmitters." This is directly beneficial to many mental health concerns. A major depressive episode, for example, is often characterized by depletion of glutamate and GABA. Both neurotransmitters have their pathways turned on by exercise.

Not only does exercise affect blood flow and brain metabolism, it also physically changes the brain. One study shows that regular aerobic exercise creates new neurons and increases mass in the hippocampus, a part of the brain responsible for memory and thinking. In addition, when cells in the body are stressed by exercise, they release growth factors in the brain, improving the health of existing brain cells, growing new blood vessels in the brain and even improving the survival of new brain cells. Research demonstrates that exercise is protective against changes in the physical brain associated with aging, concluding that exercise is an essential part of long-term optimal brain functioning, ultimately decreasing the chances of developing age-related cognitive decline.

What you can do

You can start today. It doesn't take much, and you don't have to become fit overnight. But committing to a goal of regular exercise to get your heart rate up or your muscles engaged can be enough to support your mental health for the long term. If possible, get even more benefit by exercising outside in a green environment. Going for a walk three times a week is enough to begin to feel a change without any side effects or costs to you. If it helps, find a group of like-minded people and get moving together. This improves your mental health in the ways discussed above, and the sense of community, companionship and friendship also has a beneficial impact on mood.

Ultimately, I think—and research shows—that exercise is an important component in mental health. A yin/yang approach helps to create balance with exercise. By that I mean relaxing (yin) and energetic (yang) forms of exercise—for example, hatha yoga and running, or tai chi and biking. See the following table for other examples.

YIN RELAXING, TONIFYING, NOURISHING, RESTING	YANG ENERGETIC, DYNAMIC, ACTIVE, EXERTION
Yoga	Running, jogging
Stretching	Biking
Breathing exercises	Vigorous hiking
Qi gong	Squash, tennis
Tai chi	Swimming laps
Gentle gardening	CrossFit
Walking	Boxing
Gentle swimming	Dancing

REFLECTIONS FROM MY JOURNEY
....

I have been a runner for many decades. I have used exercise as an anti-depressant to manage my mood, to manage my stress and my weight, and as a meditative practice. I have competed in many races: 10K, several half-marathons, three full marathons, sprint distance triathlons, Olympic distance triathlons, half-Ironman triathlons, and a full Ironman. In my university days, I was on the varsity track team, competing at the national level. But in 2010 I got injured, was not able to run, and required knee surgery. This set me back physically, mentally, emotionally and spiritually, and I slipped into a depression. It highlighted to me how much I had relied on exercise to manage my mood and how little balance I had in this area. Today, I have more balance in my exercise routine and listen to my body by not pushing through when I have pain.

While I was bulimic, I used both food and exercise as coping mechanisms to manage stress. When I stopped purging, I still binged and exercised. If I had an extra helping of cake, I would say to myself that I would run an extra mile the next day to compensate for the additional unwanted calories I had consumed. I ended up exercising even more and was very obsessive about it. When that was pointed out to me, I purposely decided not to exercise after I had binged. I sat with my emotions the next day instead of running that extra mile. That was hard. Many emotions came up: self-hatred, frustration, angst, fear, sabotage and more questions. What would be the consequences of bingeing and not exercising? What if I did gain weight or lose my six-pack?

If you currently have an exercise regime that you love, keep it up! If you don't, I highly recommend you get started after getting your doctor's go-ahead. It is important to do exercise that you love, whether that's gardening, walking, tennis, swimming, cycling, running, skiing, hiking, or something else. I credit tennis with lifting a depression that had been weighing me down for several months in 2009. A friend asked me to play tennis, and we started playing a few nights a week. I was now engaging in a social activity with a friend, getting outside in the fresh air, getting sunlight and vitamin D and stimulating my appetite. After two months of this, I was no longer depressed!

A side benefit of exercising to support your mood is that you may lose weight. But remember that 80% of weight loss is due to diet, while only 20% is due to exercise. To put this in perspective, 45 minutes of exercise can be destroyed by five minutes of poor nutritional intake. If weight loss is your key objective, then it is best to look at what you are eating (see Chapters 10 to 13). When it comes to supporting your mood with exercise, there are three key components:

1. **Frequency:** This is defined as how many times per week you exercise. The frequency needs to be three to five times a week to manage your mood.
2. **Duration:** This is the length of time you exercise per session. It needs to be 30 to 60 minutes for mood management.
3. **Intensity:** This refers to how hard the heart works during exercise. For weight loss and mood management, it is recommended that heart rate intensity be 70% of your maximum heart rate. The way to calculate your maximum heart rate is to subtract your age from 220. For example, if you're 40 years old, subtract 40 from 220 to get a maximum heart rate of 180. This is the maximum number of times your heart should beat per minute (bpm) while you're exercising. To support one's mood and burn fat for weight loss, a heart rate of 126 bpm (70% of 180) is recommended for a 40-year-old.

Take note of your current exercise program and adjust as necessary to address the three key areas outlined above: frequency, duration and intensity. Also, incorporate a balance between yin and yang forms of exercise. Lastly, from a physical perspective, the greatest gains are made when doing both strength (i.e., lifting weights) and cardiovascular (i.e., running) forms of exercise.

Remember that exercise is an important pillar of health. It's easy to come up with objections and excuses when it comes to exercise. Nike was bang on with its slogan—"Just do it"—to help overcome them:

- Objection: I don't have time; SOLUTION: JUST DO IT
- Objection: I don't want to get sweaty; SOLUTION: JUST DO IT
- Objection: It will take too long; SOLUTION: JUST DO IT
- Objection: I don't have anyone to go with; SOLUTION: JUST DO IT
- Objection: I slept in; SOLUTION: JUST DO IT
- Objection: I just ate, so now I will get a cramp; SOLUTION: JUST DO IT

- Objection: I am out of shape; SOLUTION: JUST DO IT
- Objection: It is too hard; SOLUTION: JUST DO IT

O— *In your* **Moving Beyond** *journal, write about the beliefs and excuses you might have about exercise. Can you overcome them by making one change?*

Exercise is an inexpensive, effective and safe treatment option and needs to be included as part of a comprehensive wellness treatment plan for mental health concerns. For me, exercise is not about what kind of outfit you are wearing or how much makeup you have on while you pose at the gym. It is a meditative experience where I am one with both nature and the sound of my beating heart as they calm the "busyness" of my mind into a state of pure bliss and joy. The goal is to do something fun, that you love, that moves your body and that causes you to sweat a little. You feel better from a mood perspective, and your heart and body will be grateful too. If we as a nation participate and engage in exercising our bodies, we can work to manage the mental health concerns of our present and future society.

(16)
Environment

"The environment of the cell determines the health of the cell."
DR. CHRIS

WHAT DO YOUR Teflon frying pan, microwave popcorn, pizza box and lipstick have in common? How about a receipt from the store, a can of tuna and a plastic water bottle? Let's not forget that cute rubber duck in the bathtub, anti-bacterial hand soap near the sink, and the Colgate Total toothpaste and deodorant in the bathroom cabinet. The answer is chemicals—namely, perfluorooctanoic acid (PFOA), bisphenol A (BPA), mercury, triclosan and phthalates. According to the Canadian authors of *Slow Death by Rubber Duck: How the Toxic Chemistry of Every-day Life Affects our Health*, this is a bad news story with a positive outcome.

Sources of contamination

The bad news is that our bodies are affected daily by chemicals from environmental pollutants, medications and hormones in our food supply, cooking utensils and containers (plastic), pots and pans (Teflon and other non-stick surfaces), pesticides and chemicals in our food, chlorine and other chemical contaminants in our water supply, chemicals in cleaning products, cosmetic products (perfume, hair products, lotions and makeup), children's toys, canned foods, as well as pollutants in the air we breathe. In recent years, many studies have shown that significant levels of toxic substances can leach from the everyday items in our homes and workplaces. We are now into the fourth generation of people exposed to toxic chemicals from before conception through to adulthood, and statistics tell us that we are under siege. The cumulative effect of these chemicals can affect our mental health, contributing to ADHD, depression and dementia. In addition, these chemicals contribute to a wide variety of health concerns, including reproductive problems, hormone imbalances, breast cancer, testicular cancer, fatigue, immune dysfunction, asthma, birth defects and liver damage.

Some of the chemicals mentioned above have a short life in the body, but others are persistent—which is a problem not only for you as an individual, but for the planet. However, it is not all a doom and gloom story. As the toxic load in our bodies continues to increase, detoxification is critical to maintain optimal health. The first steps are:

1. Understand your body's natural detoxification processes (see Chapter 13).
2. Learn what factors in our everyday lives disrupt this process (complete the Environmental Quiz on the opposite page).
3. Take the necessary steps to get back on track. This includes a carefully designed nutritional detoxification program that is supported by research and science.

Ideally, the body should be able to detoxify itself. But keep in mind that your body's ability to detoxify may be impaired by such factors as prescription medications, constipation, poor kidney health, insufficient detoxifying enzymes, poor liver health, or insufficient quantities of the nutrients, vitamins and minerals that the liver and other detoxification systems need to perform effectively. Our bodies weren't designed to cope with the level of toxins we are exposed to now.

Toxicity is a becoming a health crisis. We ingest new chemicals, use more medication, eat more sugar and refined foods and abuse ourselves daily with various stimulants or sedatives. The incidence of many toxicity-induced diseases has increased as well. In addition to anxiety and depression, many people suffer from ongoing fatigue, bloating, headaches, pain, skin irritations and constant colds and coughs. The role the environment plays in your health cannot be ignored.

A common explanation when it comes to depression and anxiety is that you aren't making enough of the neurotransmitter serotonin, so you need a medication to increase the amount of it in your brain. Selective serotonin reuptake inhibitors (SSRIs) are commonly prescribed. These include citalopram (Celexa), escitalopram (Cipralex), fluoxetine (Prozac), fluvoxamine (Luvox), Paroxetine (Paxil) and sertraline (Zoloft).

As the name SSRI implies, these medications block serotonin from being reabsorbed by the releasing cell so that more is available to bind to the next neuron in the brain. As serotonin builds up, normal communication between cells can return and symptoms of depression may improve. The entire premise behind SSRIs is that you have a deficiency problem and aren't making enough serotonin.

However, what if that is not the case? What if you are making enough serotonin, but the serotonin you are making is not getting into the next cell because there are chemicals from the environment blocking the receptors? (For a helpful visual about how serotonin is made, see Chapter 10.)

Perhaps there might not be a manufacturing problem or a deficiency problem when it comes to making neurotransmitters. Traditionally, this is the party line when you speak to an MD or psychiatrist, and it may be true in some cases. But an overlooked aspect of mental well-being is the ability of the neurotransmitter, once made, to get into the cell. It is possible that chemicals from the environment are blocking or occupying your receptors so that the neurotransmitters cannot get in to do their job.

An important step is to assess your level of environmental toxicity by completing the quiz below. This quiz points out factors in our everyday lives that disrupt our natural ability to detoxify.

ENVIRONMENTAL QUIZ

Check each item that applies to you.

_____ Do you drink pop, calorie-free or sugary drinks? This includes mixing them with alcohol (for example, rum and Coke).

_____ Do you drink anything out of a plastic bottle?

_____ Do you store hot food in a plastic container or heat your food in plastic?

_____ Do you use non-stick frying pans?

_____ Do you drink vitamin mineral water?

_____ Do you use a microwave?

_____ Do you use a cell phone or a computer for more than three hours a day?

_____ Do you frequently use ibuprofen, acetaminophen, loperamide (Imodium) or any over-the-counter medication?

_____ Do you eat foods that contain food colouring (like Smarties, M&Ms, Skittles, orange cheddar cheese)?

_____ Do you consume canned goods?

_____ Do you use personal care products with phthalates or parabens?

_____ Do you drink more than two alcoholic drinks per day?

_____ Do you exercise less than 30 minutes per day, four days per week?

_____ Do you regularly consume foods that are genetically modified? *These foods include corn, soy or soybeans, canola oil, cottonseed oil and beet sugar.*

_____ Do you eat any of the following foods in their non-organic forms?

1. Strawberries
2. Spinach
3. Nectarines
4. Apples
5. Peaches
6. Pears
7. Cherries
8. Grapes
9. Celery
10. Tomatoes
11. Bell peppers
12. Potatoes

These are the foods that are the most heavily sprayed with chemicals, according to the Environmental Working Group.

_____ Do you drink manufactured orange juice?

_____ Do you suffer from any of the following: ongoing fatigue, headaches, pain, constant colds and coughs?

_____ Do you regularly experience digestive concerns, such as gas, bloating, constipation, diarrhea or irritable bowel syndrome?

_____ Have you been diagnosed with low thyroid function or a skin condition (such as eczema, psoriasis, acne)?

_____ Do you use hand sanitizer with triclosan or Colgate Total toothpaste on a regular basis?

_____ Are you more than 15 pounds overweight?

_____ Do you wear perfume or cologne?

Score: _____

REVIEW YOUR SCORE

Less than 5

You win top marks and qualify for the "Squeaky Clean" award—congrats!

Between 5 and 12

You need an integrated detoxification program. Schedule an appointment with a naturopathic doctor today!

Greater than 12

It is time to make some serious changes to support your body. Consult with a naturopathic doctor today, as you are critically in need of care.

If you scored higher than 5, look at what you checked off and see what areas you can make changes in.

- Can you commit to eating foods that aren't genetically modified?
- Can you stop drinking water out of plastic water bottles?
- Can you stop storing or heating food in plastic containers?

O━ *Take the time to do the Environmental Quiz. In your **Moving Beyond** journal, list the steps you can take to decrease your environmental body burden.*

Understanding toxins

Here are brief explanations of why some of the items mentioned in the Environmental Quiz are unhealthy for you.

1. **Full-sugar soft drinks and diet soft drinks.** It is well recognized that sugary soft drinks are unhealthy for many reasons—they increase overall calorie intake, they create inflammation in the body and they disrupt proper insulin levels. It is also recognized that sugar-free and diet soft drinks containing aspartame may be just as dangerous for our health as full-sugar soft drinks.
    - *Solution*: Cut down or eliminate full-sugar and diet soft drinks from your diet.

2. **BPA-containing bottles and containers.** Bisphenol A (BPA), a chemical present in most plastics and tin can linings, is a known endocrine disruptor and has been linked with negative birth outcomes, infertility, thyroid dysfunction, cancer, obesity and insulin resistance.
    - *Solution:* Reduce your exposure by using stainless steel or glass water bottles, buying products and canned food packaged with BPA-free liners, using glass containers to store food, and using activated charcoal filters for drinking water. A few companies, such as Eden Organics, sell cans lined with non-BPA alternatives.

3. **Other plastic containers.** When heated, plastics begin to break down, releasing harmful chemicals into food and liquids.
    - *Solution:* Use glass or lead-free ceramic containers to reheat food in the oven or heat food on the stovetop, replace plastic containers with glass, and don't let plastic wrap touch hot food.

4. **Non-stick frying pans.** For decades, non-stick frying pans have been coated with polytetrafluoroethylene (PTFE), otherwise known as Teflon. It has been shown that when heated, Teflon releases toxic fumes that can kills birds and cause humans to have flu-like symptoms.
    - *Solution:* Use cast-iron, stainless steel or ceramic frying pans.

5. **Vitamin mineral water.** Many are loaded with sugar, and some use sweeteners or fructose, which are known to disrupt sugar metabolism, alter blood sugar levels and contribute to diabetes and weight gain.
    - *Solution:* Drink water instead. Add fresh lemon, orange or cucumber slices if you need flavour.

6. **Microwave use.** Microwaves emit a form of non-ionizing radiation (as opposed to X-rays) that vibrates water molecules to create heat. While they are under strict manufacturing regulation to minimize

human exposure, older and dirty microwaves and aging door seals can allow for large radiation leakage.

- *Solution:* Heat foods and liquids on the stovetop or in the oven; if using a microwave, check door seal for safety and stand at least 1.5 metres away while it is on.

7. **Cell phone use (> 3hrs/day).** Computers and cell phones emit non-ionizing radiation into the body and cause DNA damage.
   - *Solution:* Minimize your use of mobile phones and take frequent breaks from computer use.

8. **Artificial colouring in foods.** Studies have linked artificial colouring in foods with ADHD behaviour in children and with an increased risk of cancer in the entire population.
   - *Solution:* Avoid foods containing artificial colouring.

9. **Cosmetic products with parabens.** Parabens can mimic estrogen and have been detected in human breast cancer tissues, suggesting a possible association between parabens in cosmetics and cancer.
   - *Solution:* Use paraben-free personal care products.

10. **Perfume and fragrances.** Although you may be diligent about reading ingredient lists, phthalates are often not listed. The word "fragrance" or "parfum" near the end of the ingredient list is your clue that the product contains phthalates. Phthalates have been linked with asthma, ADHD, breast cancer, autism spectrum disorders, obesity, type 2 diabetes, altered reproductive development and male infertility
    - *Solution:* Avoid products that contain artificial fragrance or perfume; opt for essential oils instead.

11. **Genetically modified foods.** Despite much controversy over the safety of GMO foods, the truth is that we don't have enough research to deem them safe for human consumption.
    - *Solution:* Limit your consumption of the most commonly modified foods: corn, soy, canola, cottonseed oil and beet sugar.

12. **Pesticides and other food sprays.** Some of the most common synthetic pesticides, such as organophosphates and glycol ethers, have been identified as endocrine disruptors, and many contain ingredients known to increase the risk of cancer, reproductive difficulties and neurological diseases. Pesticides also damage the environment

where they are used, reaching dangerous concentrations in the soil and killing local ecosystem life.

- *Solution:* Start with the Dirty Dozen, the 12 fruits and vegetables most heavily sprayed with pesticides. Buy organic varieties of these. If you can't, then try to stick to the Clean Fifteen, the least-sprayed produce. See lists on pages 191–192.

13. **Manufactured orange juice.** Most store-bought orange juice is so heavily processed that it is barely orange juice anymore. Once oranges are pressed, the juice can be stored up to a year. Oxygen is removed from the storage tanks to keep the juice from going bad. The flavour is lost in this process, and is restored by synthetic compounds.
    - *Solution:* Juice your own oranges. Keep the pulp for the added benefit of fibre.

14. **Anti-bacterial soap and toothpastes with triclosan.** Triclosan, a chemical commonly used in some types of disinfectants soap and toothpaste, is known to interfere with a natural detoxification process in the liver that helps flush toxins from the body. The FDA has recognized that anti-bacterial products may also be contributing to widespread antibiotic resistance.
    - *Solution:* Avoid anti-bacterial soaps and ensure your toothpaste does not contain triclosan.

15. **Alcohol.** As few as two drinks a day can increase a woman's risk of developing breast cancer by as much as 41%. This points to the large role that alcohol plays in hormonal dysregulation due to its effect on the liver.
    - *Solution:* Men should limit drinks to no more than 1 or 2 per day, and women no more than 1.

16. **Ibuprofen, acetaminophen and other over-the-counter (OTC) medications.** Many use OTC medications on a regular basis. It's important to remember that simply because it's available without consulting a doctor doesn't mean it's always safe. There can be both acute and chronic risks with OTC medications.
    - *Solution:* Listen to your body. Consult with a naturopathic doctor, who can determine the root cause of your health concerns and reduce the need to use OTC medication.

17. **Excess weight.** Extra weight is a storehouse for chemicals and other factors that dysregulate hormones.
    - *Solution:* Eat a nutritious diet, exercise regularly and maintain a healthy weight.

The Dirty Dozen

The Environmental Working Group produces the Dirty Dozen list annually. It's a list of the most heavily sprayed produce. It's best to eat organic versions of these or grow them yourself. There is also a list of the Clean Fifteen—foods that are not heavily sprayed with chemicals. If finances are an issue, these are foods that you don't need to buy organic. Choosing organic foods when possible is a positive step, not only for your own health but for the planet's, as it helps reduce the quantity of chemicals sprayed in the environment.

PRODUCE WITH THE HIGHEST LEVELS OF PESTICIDES

2017 DIRTY DOZEN

1.	Strawberries	7.	Cherries
2.	Spinach	8.	Grapes
3.	Nectarines	9.	Celery
4.	Apples	10.	Tomatoes
5.	Peaches	11.	Sweet bell peppers
6.	Pears	12.	Potatoes

PRODUCE WITH THE LOWEST LEVELS OF PESTICIDES

2017 CLEAN FIFTEEN

1. Sweet corn
2. Avocado
3. Pineapple
4. Cabbage
5. Onions
6. Sweet peas frozen
7. Papaya*
8. Asparagus
9. Mangoes
10. Eggplant
11. Honeydew melon
12. Kiwi
13. Cantaloupe
14. Cauliflower
15. Grapefruit

* A small amount of sweet corn, papaya and summer squash sold in the United States is produced from genetically modified seeds. Buy organic varieties of these crops if you want to avoid genetically modified produce.

In addition to the Dirty Dozen and Clean Fifteen lists, the Environmental Working Group also has a Dirty Dozen list of endocrine disruptors. There is no end to the tricks that endocrine disruptors can play on our bodies:

- Increasing production of certain hormones
- Decreasing production of others
- Imitating hormones
- Turning one hormone into another
- Interfering with hormone signalling
- Telling cells to die prematurely
- Competing with essential nutrients
- Binding to essential hormones
- Accumulating in cells that produce hormones

These imbalances contribute to sleep disorders, depression, anxiety, fertility challenges, hormone imbalances, weight gain, skin problems, cancers and much more. See the Appendix for a list of endocrine hormone disruptors, how they affect your hormones and how to avoid them.

In previous chapters, the importance of digestive health and liver function was discussed. It is important to recognize that there is a correlation between depression and anxiety and poor diet and low nutrition. Many people's bodies are overloaded with toxins from their diet and the environment. Also, eating too much sugar leads to an overgrowth of bad bacteria and candida in the digestive system.

As discussed in Chapter 13, a good detox is not just about cleansing the liver. It is about correcting the diet, addressing environmental toxins in your environment, removing bad bacteria, re-populating the gut with healthy organisms, rebalancing pH levels, ensuring the kidneys are working effectively, and supporting the drainage and detoxification processes of the liver. This is known as an integrated detoxification. To get the best results, it is important that such a cleanse be supervised by your naturopathic doctor so that concerns can be addressed as they arise. It is also important to ensure you are completing the detoxification steps in the right order. Often, this approach results in significant improvement in your overall well-being.

A key step that most people miss in detoxification is eliminating your exposure to environmental toxins in the first place. A good resource on this subject is *Clean, Green, and Lean: Get Rid of the Toxins That Make You Fat,* by Dr. Walter Crinnion.

Protecting yourself

While the Environmental Quiz is fun to do and gives you an idea of the areas you need to change, more objective tests are available through naturopathic doctors to assess the levels of heavy metals, environmental pollutants, solvents/volatile organic compounds (VOCs), BPA, triclosan, 4-nonylphenol, parabens and phthalates in your body. Based on the results, an individualized treatment program can be customized to support your organs of detoxification, which include your liver, kidneys, colon, lungs, skin and lymphatic system. The following simple steps are also recommended to protect your family:

1. Read ingredients labels on products. Phthalates often are not listed; however, the word "fragrance" or "parfum" near the end of the ingredient list is your clue that the product usually contains phthalates.

2. Unplug air fresheners, as many contain phthalates. Baking soda is a natural alternative that can be used to absorb bad odours.

3. Visit ecocenter.org to check out ingredients in the toys you own or want to purchase to ensure they are not harmful for your children.

4. Avoid fast food. Food wrap for hamburgers, pizza and microwaveable popcorn may be coated with perfluorinated compounds (PFCs).

5. BPA leaches from containers into contents and we end up consuming it. Containers do not need to be heated for this to occur. Switch to glass or stainless steel containers where possible for storing your food. Do not microwave your leftovers in polycarbonate or plastic containers—use glass instead. Do not use a plastic lid cover in the microwave. Better yet, don't use a microwave.

6. Change cookware from non-stick or Teflon (especially if scratched) to stainless steel, ceramic or cast-iron. Change plastic cooking spoons and spatulas to wood or metal.

7. Buy flaked, skipjack or chunk light tuna instead of solid white (albacore) tuna, which has the highest levels of mercury. King mackerel, shark, swordfish and tilefish also contain high levels of mercury, so avoid these as well. (See the mercury fish list on page 195.)

8. Avoid products labelled "anti-bacterial" that contain triclosan (e.g., Microban). Wash your hands the "old-fashioned" way, with a good 30-second lather of soap and water. Note: Colgate Total toothpaste also contains triclosan.

9. Check out the Environmental Working Group's Cosmetic Database to find out what's in your cosmetics. If your products rate greater than 5 out of 10 on the toxicity scale, find healthier alternatives by visiting a health food store.

10. When puzzling over the small recycling numbers on the bottoms of plastic containers, remember this mnemonic: 4, 5, 1 and 2; all the rest are bad for you.

11. Use cloth or paper bags instead of plastic bags for shopping.

12. Encourage politicians to introduce legislation to phase out PFCs from food wrappers and other consumer products and to legislate for better control of triclosan. Demand non-toxic toys for your children.

Mercury in fish

MOST TOXIC (Parts per million)	LEAST TOXIC (Parts per million)
1. Tilefish (Gulf of Mex) **1.45**	1. Scallop **0.0003**
2. Swordfish **0.995**	2. Canned Salmon **0.008**
3. Shark **0.979**	3. Clam **0.009**
4. King Mackerel **0.73**	4. Shrimp **0.009**
5. Tuna (Bigeye) Fresh/Frozen **0.689**	5. Oyster **0.012**
6. Orange Roughy **0.571**	6. Tilapia **0.013**
7. Marlin **0.485**	7. Sardine **0.013**
8. Mackerel Spanish (Gulf of Mex) **0.454**	8. Anchovies **0.017**
9. Grouper **0.448**	9. Salmon Fresh/Frozen **0.022**
10. Tuna Fresh/Frozen **0.415**	10. Squid **0.023**
11. Bluefish **0.368**	11. Catfish **0.025**
12. Sablefish **0.361**	12. Pollock **0.031**
13. Chilean Bass **0.354**	13. Crawfish **0.033**
14. White Croaker (Pacific) **0.287**	14. Shad American **0.045**
15. Halibut **0.241**	15. Atlantic Mackerel **0.05**
16. Weakfish (Sea Trout) **0.235**	16. Mullet **0.05**
17. Scorpion Fish **0.233**	17. Whiting **0.051**
18. Lobster **0.166**	18. Haddock (Atlantic) **0.055**
19. Snapper **0.166**	19. Flatfish **0.056**
20. Bass (Saltwater, Black) **0.152**	20. Butterfish **0.058**
	SOURCE: U.S. Food and Drug Administration

13. Refer to the Environmental Working Group's Dirty Dozen and Clean Fifteen lists annually to see which fruits and vegetables contain the greatest and smallest levels of pesticides.

14. Use fresh fruits and vegetables instead of canned whenever possible, particularly if you are pregnant. Alternatively, select products that are packaged in glass or cardboard containers, or that have been frozen when fresh. If you do use canned foods, look for products labelled BPA-free. A few companies, such as Eden Organics, provide canned products lined with non-BPA alternatives.

15. With respect to baby formula, choose powdered formula because the packaging contains less BPA. If your baby needs liquid formula, look for brands sold in non-plastic containers.

16. Watch receipts. In 2010, the Environmental Working Group tested retailers' store receipts and found that 40% were coated with BPA. This chemical can rub off on your hands or food items. Some may be absorbed through the skin. Limit your exposure by: 1) saying no to receipts when possible; 2) keeping receipts in an envelope; 3) never giving a child a receipt to hold or play with; 4) washing your hands before preparing and eating food after handling receipts; and 5) not recycling receipts and other thermal paper, so BPA residues will not contaminate recycled paper.

When we compare our modern-day lives with those of our grandparents, it is clear that our environment has changed greatly. We are exposed to hundreds of times more chemicals, toxins, and different forms of radiation than generations past. At the same time, chronic disease rates are soaring. The quality of the air you breathe, the food you eat, the water you drink and the chemicals your skin is exposed to matter and add up quickly. Your health depends on your ability to decrease your exposure to harmful chemicals. Also, how well your detoxification organs break down and eliminate chemicals plays a crucial role in supporting your overall health, including your mental health. The good news is that with greater awareness and by encouraging change, you will be helping not only your individual health but the collective health of your community and this great planet we all call home.

(17)

A Word About Stress

*"With awareness of faulty beliefs in the present moment,
we can change our future behaviour."*

DR. CHRIS

THE WORD "STRESS" is frequently used in our culture to describe a wide variety of situations—from sitting in rush hour traffic, to the feelings associated with intense demands from your boss, to going through a difficult divorce or losing your job. "Stress" is such a common word today that it's hard to believe the current use of the term originated only 50 years ago.

The term came about because of pioneering research conducted by Dr. Hans Seyle, a Canadian endocrinologist. Dr. Seyle made a distinction between the terms "stress" and "stressor." A stressor is an actual or perceived source of danger that activates the stress response mechanism. Stress is the physiological response to the stressor. In the past, stressors were short-lived—such as being chased by a lion in the hunter-gatherer days. Today, people refer to having a certain amount of stress in their lives, but what they are really referring to is a certain number of stressors.

This is an important distinction to make, as it is helpful when it comes to managing stress reduction. In our go-go society, it feels like we have a constant input of stressors; our foot is always on the gas pedal. It is important to develop your awareness of what stress means to you as an individual. Everyone's capacity to handle stress is different, and it is important not to compare yourself with anyone else.

Stress is the response of the body and spirit to any demand. Any demand made upon us in the course of a day brings about certain reactions in the body. Our ability to cope with the demands upon us is key to our experience of stress. For example, starting a new job might be an exciting experience if everything else in your life is stable and positive. But if you start a new job when you've just moved into a new house in a new city, or your partner is ill, or you're experiencing money problems, then you might find it harder to cope.

It is helpful to understand that there are many different types of stress:

TYPE OF STRESS	EXAMPLE
Physical/physiological	Surgery or chronic disease
Emotional	Divorce, death of a loved one
Mental	Work, school
Psychological	Any negative thought patterns that are not serving you positively
Life	Any significant change, such as moving or negotiating with difficult teenagers

How many stressors can you handle? Some life events are easier to deal with than others. For example, compare the intensity of getting divorced with that of a change in responsibilities at work. To get the complete picture, you need to be able to rate and measure stressors appropriately. The Social Readjustment Rating Scale, more commonly known as the Holmes and Rahe Stress Scale, was created to do just that.

This scale is a well-known tool for measuring the number of stressors you've experienced within the past year. Taking the test can help you see clearly if you're at risk of illness due to too many stressors, as it helps measure the stress load you carry. Take some time now to do the inventory for yourself.

THE HOLMES AND RAHE STRESS SCALE

To score your stress levels, simply answer Yes or No to the statements below depending on whether they have happened to you in the last year.

1.	Death of spouse (100)	Yes	No
2.	Divorce (73)	Yes	No
3.	Marital separation (65)	Yes	No
4.	Jail term (63)	Yes	No
5.	Death of close family member (63)	Yes	No
6.	Personal injury or illness (53)	Yes	No
7.	Marriage (50)	Yes	No
8.	Fired at work (47)	Yes	No
9.	Marital reconciliation (45)	Yes	No
10.	Retirement (45)	Yes	No
11.	Change in health of family member (44)	Yes	No
12.	Pregnancy (40)	Yes	No
13.	Sex difficulties (39)	Yes	No
14.	Gain of new family member (39)	Yes	No
15.	Business readjustment (39)	Yes	No
16.	Change in financial state (38)	Yes	No
17.	Death of close friend (37)	Yes	No
18.	Change to a different line of work (36)	Yes	No
19.	Change in number of arguments with spouse (35)	Yes	No
20.	A large mortgage or loan (30)	Yes	No
21.	Foreclosure of mortgage or loan (30)	Yes	No
22.	Change in responsibilities at work (29)	Yes	No
23.	Son or daughter leaving home (29)	Yes	No
24.	Trouble with in-laws (29)	Yes	No
25.	Outstanding personal achievement (28)	Yes	No
26.	Spouse begins or stops work (26)	Yes	No
27.	Begin or end school/college (26)	Yes	No
28.	Change in living conditions (25)	Yes	No
29.	Revision of personal habits (24)	Yes	No
30.	Trouble with boss (23)	Yes	No
31.	Change in work hours or conditions (20)	Yes	No
32.	Change in residence (20)	Yes	No

33. Change in school/college (20)	Yes	No
34. Change in recreation (19)	Yes	No
35. Change in church activities (19)	Yes	No
36. Change in social activities (18)	Yes	No
37. A moderate loan or mortgage (37)	Yes	No
38. Change in sleeping habits (16)	Yes	No
39. Change in number of family get-togethers (15)	Yes	No
40. Change in eating habits (15)	Yes	No
41. Vacation (13)	Yes	No
42. Christmas (12)	Yes	No
43. Minor violations of the law (11)	Yes	No

SCORE INTERPRETATION

Score	Comment
11–149	You have only a low to moderate chance of becoming ill in the near future.
150–299	You have a moderate to high chance of becoming ill in the near future.
300–600	You have a high or very high risk of becoming ill in the near future.

What you can do about stress

If you find that you are at moderate or high risk, then an obvious first thing to do is to try to avoid future life crises.

While this is clearly easier said than done, you can usually avoid moving house, for example, close to when you retire, or when one of your children goes off to college; you can learn conflict resolution and non-violent communication skills to minimize conflict with other people; you can avoid taking on new obligations or engaging with new programs of study; and you can generally take things easy, and look after yourself.

Stress has physiological manifestations

One of the difficulties with stress is that the body can't differentiate between "good" and "bad" stressors. In our minds, we make a distinction between the pain caused by the loss of a loved one and the pain caused by stubbing one's toe. But the nature of the demand is unimportant at the biological and physiological levels. To the body, it's all the same because the stress response is the same. The glands in our body that respond to the stress signal from our brain and nervous system are the adrenals. The adrenal glands secrete hormones (cortisol and epinephrine) that act on the nervous system to produce an increased "fight-or-flight," or sympathetic, response and decreased parasympathetic response in the body. This results in the following symptoms:

- Increased heart rate and blood pressure ("pounding heart")
- Blood redirected to muscles and heart, away from digestive tract
- Decreased activity in digestive and urinary systems
- Cold, sweaty skin
- Dilated lung bronchioles, "rapid deep breathing"
- Dilated pupils

What does the above list closely resemble? Anxiety symptoms! The correlation between stress and anxiety is real, and is due to the physiological effects caused by adrenal hormones. Back in the hunter-gatherer days, the stress response served us well, as we were physiologically wired to run from the sabre-toothed tiger. The problem is that today, our stress response is turned on constantly rather than intermittently. Eventually, this leads to the following symptoms of adrenal fatigue:

- Depression, anxiety
- Fatigue
- Lowered immune function
- Insomnia
- Digestive complaints
- Imbalanced hormones (premenstrual syndrome [PMS], cramps, difficult menopause)
- Headaches
- Inflammation
- High blood pressure

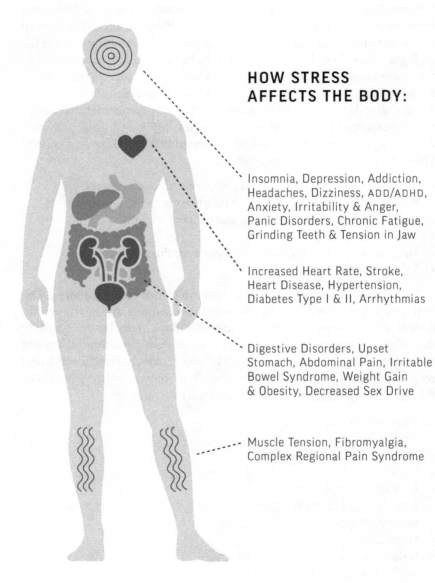

HOW STRESS
AFFECTS THE BODY:

Insomnia, Depression, Addiction, Headaches, Dizziness, ADD/ADHD, Anxiety, Irritability & Anger, Panic Disorders, Chronic Fatigue, Grinding Teeth & Tension in Jaw

Increased Heart Rate, Stroke, Heart Disease, Hypertension, Diabetes Type I & II, Arrhythmias

Digestive Disorders, Upset Stomach, Abdominal Pain, Irritable Bowel Syndrome, Weight Gain & Obesity, Decreased Sex Drive

Muscle Tension, Fibromyalgia, Complex Regional Pain Syndrome

Stress management

You know you are depleted and stress has become a problem for you when daily tasks cause you to be reactive. What can you do about it? The first step in managing stress is being aware of what is causing it and, if possible, removing it. If you can't remove the stressor, then you have to learn how to manage your reaction to what is going on in your life. Historically, the stress response was designed to respond to a physical danger, but in our modern times, it has become a response for anxiety, upset or tension in which no physical danger is present. Since we want to avoid associating stress as an emotional state, an effective strategy for situations in which anxiety, upset or tension triggers the fight-or-flight response is to create a separation between the physical stress response and the emotional response.

This is possible using the Seven Rs of working with problematic thoughts and breaking the thought–emotion cycle (see Chapter 18). This approach is helpful for addressing trauma, in which a past event triggers the stress response and now all current situations that remotely resemble the past event also trigger the stress response. By separating the stress response, one learns to interpret the present situation based on what is occurring in the moment rather than basing it on what happened in the past. By practising relaxation techniques daily, you can restore function to your neuroendocrine system. Relaxation techniques include yoga, gentle exercise (such as swimming, biking, tennis, skiing, walking), tai chi, qi gong, cooking, watching movies, journalling, doing crafts, gardening, playing music, or whatever you find soothing. Useful reference books on the effects of stress on our health include:

- *When the Body Says No: The Cost of Hidden Stress* by Dr. Gabor Maté
- *Why Zebras Don't Get Ulcers* by Robert Sapolsky
- *The Stress of Life* by Dr. Hans Selye

 ⚷ *Take the stress quiz on page 199. Write in your **Moving Beyond** journal about what is causing you stress. What are some solutions you can take to improve your situation?*

Other important steps include getting enough sleep and having a well-balanced and nourishing diet. Please refer to previous chapters for a discussion on sleep and diet. By following the advice set out in this book, you will be able to manage the curveballs life throws you, since you will have built your health on a solid foundation. In the next few chapters, we will look at how to manage your mind as it relates to stress.

(18)

Breaking the Thought–
Emotion Cycle

*"When you are stuck, what are the thoughts you are believing?
Do you need them?"*

DR. CHRIS

ONE OF THE most important areas to address when regaining your mental health is learning to identify when you get hooked, triggered or stuck in thoughts that aren't serving you. "Monkey mind" is a Buddhist term that refers to how the mind can jump around to different thoughts and states, such as being unsettled, restless, anxious, whimsical, fearful, confused, indecisive or uncontrollable. More than 2,500 years ago, Buddha taught people about the human mind so they might better understand themselves and discover that there was a way out of suffering. In my own case, I have found that learning to manage my mind has been a key to recovering my mental health.

There are many different types of psychologists and schools of thought regarding therapy, and many books written on the subject. I have taken many self-help courses, read many books, and obtained additional training in five forms of therapy: Gestalt psychotherapy, cognitive behavioural therapy (CBT), compassion-focused therapy, mindfulness-based therapy, and integrative reprogramming technique (IRT). I have compiled a list of the resources that I have found helpful; I recommend reading those that resonate with you (see Bibliography & Recommended Reading).

REFLECTIONS FROM MY JOURNEY

When I was first diagnosed with bulimia, anxiety, depression and bipolar disorder, I was not open to the idea that my thoughts played a role in how I was feeling or affected my mood. In fact, if you had suggested to me that all I needed to do was "think positive," I probably would have rolled my eyes at you and walked out of the room. I think this was because I felt that telling me to be positive implied that I was willfully choosing to be depressed—as if it was completely in my locus of control to regulate my mood by magically turning a switch on or off. What I have come to learn is that negative thinking is a *symptom* of depression. It is what depression does *to* you. It blocks your judgment and takes away your ability to remember that the sun is hiding behind the clouds. But you can learn to trip the switch by detaching from your thoughts. As it turns out, the switch is *influenced by* your thoughts—or to put it another way, by you not attaching to your thoughts.

What I teach patients is the framework outlined below on how to work with problematic thoughts and break the thought–emotion cycle. I encourage them to step out of the label they have been given and simply accept that they have a "thought pathology," or a problem with the way they have been thinking. It is important to recognize that our thought patterns get us into lots of trouble! Thoughts have a super-power "stickiness" that keeps our mind stuck around certain issues, beliefs or concepts. Once our minds are stuck, the urge to follow these thought patterns is powerful—but it doesn't lead anywhere good.

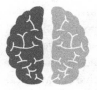 In our society, many people are either right- or left-brained in their thinking, with little crossover. This can make us unbalanced. We end up living from the neck up, stuck in our heads, with little regard for our bodies.

If you contrast this with Eastern philosophy and the yin-yang symbol in traditional Chinese medicine, you can see there is crossover in the two energy systems (i.e., there is a little yin within the yang and a little yang within the yin). The word that best describes what this symbol represents is "balance." It is this crossover that creates the harmony or balance. The difference between Eastern philosophy and Western society is that in the West, there is no crossover or balance when it comes to our "thinking" minds.

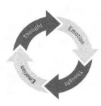

Because of our "thinking minds," we remain stuck in our heads with thoughts that trigger an emotion, which triggers another thought, which triggers an emotion, and round and round we go. Most people remain stuck in depression, anxiety, anger, obsession, addiction, suicidal thoughts, stress, mania, psychosis, eating disorders and fear. In Western society, most of us are living from the neck up. We are completely stuck in our heads with our thoughts, and we become afraid of our emotions. We become possessed by the thinking mind and stuck in the thought–emotion cycle rut.

The following questions then arise: How do we break this cycle? How can we become emotionally free and not at the mercy of our thoughts? Can we even become emotionally free? Thankfully, yes, using a mind-body-spirit approach to medicine (i.e., naturopathic medicine).

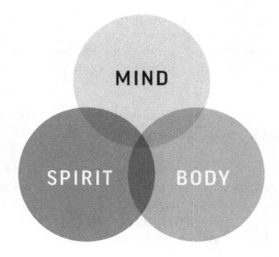

"Mind" is another word for where we hold our thoughts; "body" is another word for where we feel our emotions; and spirit is what is necessary to break the thought–emotion cycle. We need to *breathe* deeply to calm our minds and create a "space" or "gap" in our thoughts. It has been said that music is not about the notes, it is about the space between the notes. It is similar with our mind. The more space you can create between the chain reaction of your thoughts and emotions, the calmer the emotional waves of your life will be. We need to sit in our emotions and allow them to come up without any thought or judgment from our mind.

So how do we do this? The Seven Rs comprise a framework for how to work with our minds to free ourselves from the urge to follow destructive thought patterns. I was initially taught a version of this by my naturopathic doctor, Dr. Jason Hughes, to whom I owe much of the credit for teaching me how to regain my mental health by managing my mind. The Seven Rs are:

- **Recognize:** Recognize your thoughts
- **Refrain:** Refrain from following your thoughts
- **Relax:** Relax into your breath
- **Resolve:** Resolve to repeat this process
- **Rephrase/reaffirm:** Rephrase the thought you recognized
- **Reflect:** Reflect on why you have ended up unwell
- **Reward:** Reward yourself

Step 1: Recognize your thoughts

In order to change our mood, we have to have some awareness about our thoughts, when our minds go "off" and how our thoughts affect how we feel.

REFLECTIONS FROM MY JOURNEY

When I was "stuck" in depression and anxiety, I had a really hard time looking at my thoughts because I was so deeply entrenched in them. When depression and anxiety would lift, I realized that "stinking thinking" is part of the pathology picture of mental illness. It is what depression and anxiety does *to* you, but this is not who you are. I have come to realize that underneath that cloud or veil of self-doubt, there is an inherent disposition in most people to either view the world as "the cup is half empty" or "the cup is half full."

I understand how hard it is to believe that your thoughts affect your physiology and how you feel. Believe me, I was skeptical once too—I used to cringe when people would impart Louise Hay's mantra "Change your thoughts, change your life" on me. I also had a hard time accepting that there was anything I could do to change my thoughts. Whenever anyone said, "Just think positive!" or "Snap out of it," I felt like it was my fault for being depressed. I would take it personally. It made me feel as though how I was feeling was all in my head, and all I had to do was "snap out of it" and, boom, the way I was feeling would be over. I used to believe that saying those words to someone who is depressed was akin to asking a blind person to see or a deaf person to hear. So, trust me—I know how hard it is to hear suggestions like these when you are depressed. I also know that a lack of insight into how you are thinking may limit you in regaining your mental health.

The beautiful thing is that you can change how you view the world. You are not fixed in any way, shape or form. This is the concept of neuroplasticity. Essentially, your brain has a plastic, or bendy, quality to it and can change. You can create new neural pathways in your brain, essentially rewiring it to think in a new way. And if your thoughts reflect a new way of being, then you can affect your entire physiology because your thoughts affect neuropeptides. Neuropeptides are signalling molecules that influence brain and body activities. They bind to receptors and affect how your body functions. Neuropeptides are involved in a variety of brain functions, including pain management, reward, food intake, metabolism, reproduction, social behaviours, learning and more. This idea stems from the work of Dr. Candace Pert and the field of psychoneuroimmunology (PNI). PNI is a big word that, when broken down, means:

- psycho = thoughts
- neuro = brain
- immunology = immune system

The takeaway points from this research are: 1) your subconscious and conscious beliefs are important components to your health; 2) thoughts create neuropeptides, which bind to receptors in our brain and body, influencing our physiology. I want to be clear here: I am not saying that if you are anxious or depressed, you have caused it yourself with your thinking. I am, however, saying that if you can gain insight into what you are thinking and, most importantly, bring compassion and love to yourself, then the seeds of recovery can be planted. We must be careful how we are talking to ourselves because not only are we listening, but our thoughts are affecting our physiology, based on PNI research. I find this passage from Anita Moorjani's book *Dying to Be Me* extremely helpful.

> Sweeping statements such as 'Negative thoughts attract negativity in life' aren't necessarily true, and can make people who are going through a challenging time feel even worse. It can also create fear that they're going to attract even more negativity with their thoughts. Using this idea indiscriminately often makes people going through seemingly tough times feel as though they're bad for attracting such events, and that's just not true. If we start to believe that it's our negative thoughts that are creating any unpleasant situations, we can become paranoid about what we're thinking. On the contrary, it actually has less to do with our thoughts than with our emotions, especially what we feel about ourselves...I can't say this strongly enough, but our feelings about ourselves are actually the most important barometer for determining the condition of our lives! In other words, being true to ourselves is more important than just trying to stay positive!
>
> I allow myself to feel negatively about things that upset me because it's much better to experience real emotions than to bottle them up. Once again, it's about allowing what I'm actually feeling, rather than fighting against it. The very act of permitting without judgment is an act of self-love. This act of kindness toward myself goes much further in creating a joyful life than falsely pretending to feel optimistic.

Loving and accepting ourselves is a critical component to regaining our mental health. When you learn to love and accept yourself, you think differently about yourself. And if you think differently about yourself, you will no longer be at war with yourself. You may be free from the thoughts of depression and anxiety that plague you. You can change your thoughts and your life will change. If you are to truly recover or be cured from mental dis-ease, this is a must. I have found, however, in working with many patients, that it is much easier to incorporate this step when you have permanently cemented the physical foundation addressed in the previous chapters regarding diet, nutrition and supplementation; stress awareness; sleep; and exercise.

Recognizing your thoughts is a critical step. And what you must recognize is that you are stuck! A useful quote by Eckhart Tolle that can help is: "The emotions are our bodies' reaction to thought. Emotion arises at the place where mind and body meet. It is the body's reaction to your mind. Or you might say, a reflection of your mind in the body." Chances are if you are *feeling* strong emotions, you are probably "stuck" somewhere. Start paying attention to what is going on inside your head. If what you are thinking is unkind, unsupportive, destructive, mean, unhelpful, negative, based in fear, defeatist or anything along that vein, then you are stuck. Move on to Step 2.

Step 2: Refrain from following your thoughts

Once you have awareness about *how* you are thinking, then the next step is to refrain from following thoughts that contribute to a negative mood state or perpetuate fear and anxiety in the body. Often these thoughts fuel the seeds of self-doubt, self-hatred and criticism. These seeds end up growing like uncontrollable weeds that take over and destroy the garden of our minds. Ultimately, we want to get to the point where these seeds are not even planted. We want to pluck all the weeds out of our minds, so they can't reproduce, and replace them with fruitful thoughts. Because these thinking patterns run deep into your history, it is crucial to master this step and refrain from following the urge to perpetuate destructive thinking patterns. A useful analogy here is to imagine you have a skin condition, like scabies, that makes your skin extremely itchy. All you want to do is scratch; that is all you can think about and do. The breakthrough is when you feel the itch is there and instead of scratching until it bleeds, you successfully refrain from scratching. It is like this with our thinking patterns. We get immersed in them and we follow them. The goal of refraining is to relax into the urge, into the pattern you have of wanting to follow your thoughts. The best way to help you refrain from following your thoughts is by moving on to Step 3: Relax.

Step 3: Relax

Once we refrain from our habitual "urge" to follow our thoughts, we may find that the *feeling* of being stuck is still there. This is normal. Using your breath, relax into the feeling of being "stuck" and allow yourself to feel whatever emotions may be lurking behind the thoughts. You will find that if you allow yourself to relax, both the feeling and the urge to follow your habitual responses will dissipate and lessen over time.

One of the tickets to emotional freedom lies in breaking the thought–emotion cycle. The key is learning to get out of your mind and connect with your body. But how do you do that? Through the breath. Simply allow yourself to be guided by your breath.

BREATHING PROPERLY

In normal, quiet breathing, most people rely only on the upper portion of their lungs, using muscles to expand the upper chest wall outward while leaving the abdomen unexpanded. Using only the top parts of our lungs to breathe allows only low-volume gas exchange, and neglects our lung capacity. A proper breath that promotes more gas exchange uses the full abdomen. A "full-belly breath" is a calming, oxygenating and rejuvenating.

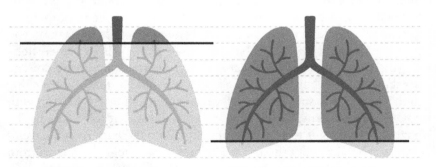

STRESS BREATHING
Shallow or Sympathetic

RELAXATION BREATHING
Deep or Parasympathetic

Just like everyone is living from the neck up, stuck in their heads in a battleground of thoughts, we are also not breathing properly; we are using only the top parts of our lungs to take shallow breaths instead of using our whole lungs to take deep breaths. Recognize that your lungs are a large organ—the fourth largest in your body. When you breathe properly, your diaphragm pulls down so your lungs can fully inflate. When the diaphragm contracts, it can tap the tops of the adrenal glands. Our adrenal glands produce stress hormones when we feel threatened or anxious. By breathing deeply, we can calm our adrenal glands and ultimately calm ourselves. If you have spent much time around someone who practises meditation or has a regular breathing, prayer or yoga practice, you may notice that they have a calm, peaceful energy about them. This is because they spend much time in quiet contemplation of their breath.

To illustrate how important breathing is, it is helpful to be reminded of first aid. If you have ever taken cardiopulmonary resuscitation (CPR), you will remember the "ABCs" of first aid:

- "A" stands for airway
- "B" stands for breathing
- "C" stands for circulation

The most important thing to check when you find someone lying comatose on the ground is their airway and breathing. Do they have an open airway? Are they breathing? This is more important than checking to see if their heart is beating. Similarly, what is the first thing obstetricians, midwives and new parents are waiting for when a baby is born? If you guessed "baby taking its first breath," you are right! Everyone is holding their breath until the newborn takes their first breath outside of the womb. And at the opposite end of our lives, when we are on our death beds, we take our last breaths before our bodies die. Breath is the gift of life. It is such a simple thing that most of us take for granted; many don't even realize they aren't breathing properly. I also think it is incredible that the Latin derivation of the word "inspire" or "inspiration" is "breathe or put life or spirit into the human body; impart reason to a human soul." To break the thought–emotion cycle, we need to learn how to breathe properly.

When you recognize that you are stuck in a negative thought pattern, a helpful way to refrain from following the thoughts any further is to relax into the breath as follows:

- Plant your feet firmly on the ground and sit up straight, focusing on the alignment of your pelvis, spine, shoulders and top of your head. Place your right hand on your belly button and your left hand on your heart (or any other part of your body that may need healing). Breathe in, slowly and deeply to a minimum count of four, through your nose into your belly so that your right hand rises by engaging your diaphragm. Exhale slowly to a minimum count of four. Breathe in again, noticing the gentle rise of your right hand as you take a proper inhalation. Exhale slowly again. As you breathe in, you can direct your focus outwards to something in nature. You can focus on the clouds, the trees, a flower or an animal. Direct your attention to see if you can see the clouds moving in the sky, the leaves of a tree moving in the wind or the different colours of a flower. By directing your attention on something outside of yourself, you shift the focus of your mind and thoughts. For a moment, when you are breathing and mindfully directing your attention, your mind will be calm and at peace. This is the goal. You will be free from thought. Take a moment to appreciate the power of pausing, creating a space or a gap between the thoughts.

- As you grow in your breathing practice, you can shift your attention to focus on the breath and allow it to gather up any tension, negativity, emotions or self-doubt that may be rocking around inside of you and send it out with the exhale. By focusing on the breath, you get out of your head and break the vicious cycle of problematic thoughts that contribute to anxiety, depression, stress, compulsive behaviours, over-eating, and other issues.

- Continue breathing for as long as you need to. Remember that this type of deep, rhythmic breathing is nature's way of calming your nervous system. Because your adrenal glands sit under your diaphragm, they can be gently massaged or calmed when you take a proper inhalation.

Here is an explanation of why you place your right hand on your belly button and your left hand over your heart:

- The right side of your body in traditional Chinese medicine (TCM) is the yang, or masculine/power, side. We want to balance our energy systems by connecting it to a yin area of our body. By placing your right hand on your belly button, you are connecting with the centre of your female energy. This is where you were once connected to your mother in her womb through the umbilical cord. It is also the location of the first and second chakras in ayurvedic medicine. In this system of medicine, our second chakra has to do with emotional regulation, our connection with ourselves and others and creativity/sexual energy. The first chakra relates to beliefs inherited during our formative years. Self-preservation, personal survival and identification with the physical world are key aspects of the first, or "root," chakra. A healthy root chakra connects you to your family of origin, which can affect your current relationships. Blockages in the second chakra relate to emotional problems, compulsive or obsessive problems, or sexual guilt; blockages in the first chakra relate to fear, procrastination, defensiveness and paranoia.

- The left side of your body in TCM is the yin, or healing/feminine/calm, side. It is important to connect the healing energy of your left hand with a part of your body that needs healing—such as your heart, stomach, head, forehead or wherever you feel, intuitively, that you need healing. If you are unsure where to place your left hand, I recommend placing it over your heart, as this represents a yang organ in TCM. By placing our right and left hands in these positions, we are balancing yin and yang. The heart is also your fourth chakra in ayurvedic medicine, connecting body and mind with spirit. In ayurvedic medicine, this is the centre for love, compassion and spirituality, and directs our ability to love ourselves and others, as well as give and receive love. Blockages in the fourth chakra relate to inhumanity, lack of compassion or unprincipled behaviour, immune dysfunction and/or lung and heart problems.

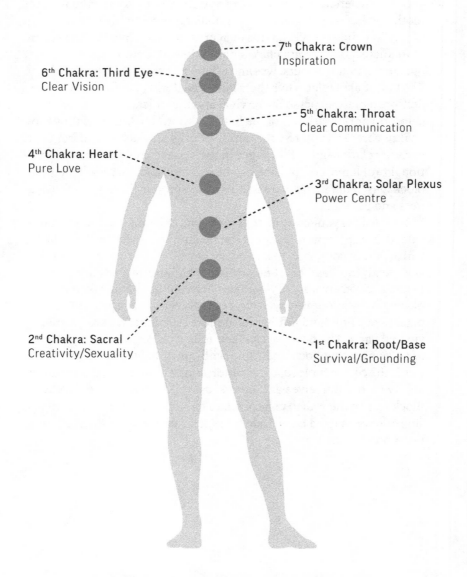

7th Chakra: Crown
Inspiration

6th Chakra: Third Eye
Clear Vision

5th Chakra: Throat
Clear Communication

4th Chakra: Heart
Pure Love

3rd Chakra: Solar Plexus
Power Centre

2nd Chakra: Sacral
Creativity/Sexuality

1st Chakra: Root/Base
Survival/Grounding

THE SEVEN CHAKRAS AND THEIR MEANINGS

The other reasons for placing your right hand on your belly button and your left hand on your heart are to:

1. Illustrate the movement of the breath through the body. If your right hand doesn't move, you know you aren't engaging your diaphragm
2. Illustrate that there are more serotonin receptors between your two hands (i.e., in your digestive tract) than in your brain
3. Illustrate that there is more electrical activity happening in your heart than in your brain

REFLECTIONS FROM MY JOURNEY

When I was first introduced to the concept of awareness and breath work, I remember feeling like I was going to be practising my breath and redirecting my attention all day long because I was so stuck in my head with negative thoughts. I was feeling depressed, suicidal and having daily attacks of anxiety, and it was very difficult to accomplish anything. The response I received from my naturopathic doctor when I told him that I would be redirecting my thoughts all day long was, "So be it." And so it was. I was practising my breath and redirecting my focus from my head to my heart. This allowed me to get out of my head and achieve a break from the tortuous thoughts that were crippling me. I often found it helpful to really look at something in nature, whether it was cloud formations, the leaves on a plant, the petals of a flower or the speckled colours in my cat's eyes. I looked as if I were seeing whatever I was looking at for the first time. This gave my mind a job to do: the job of paying attention. I added wonder, curiosity, amusement, joy and love to the mix. It took time. It took patience. It took practice. It took repetition. But eventually, change happened. Slowly, but surely. As it was for me, it will be for you too. I truly believe it will.

In essence, this step is about getting out of our heads and into our bodies and the present moment. This is why learning to have a mind–body–spirit approach to health is fundamental. The beauty of the breath is it can create a space, gap or pause in your thoughts. It can allow you to stay with whatever emotion might be rising within you, without perpetuating the cycle with another self-deprecating thought that doesn't serve you or stuffing down the energy of emotions that need to flow out of you.

When you start working with and observing your thoughts, you need to ask yourself: "Where am I living in my head?" Typically, there are three possible places:

1.   In the present moment
2.   In the past—usually ruminating about or analyzing past events
3.   In the future—often worrying about an event that hasn't happened yet.

If you tend to find yourself in the past, remind yourself that the past is over. Done. Finished. There is nothing you can do about it except change your relationship to it in the present moment. Let go, and learn and grow from the experiences you have had.

If you find you are ruminating about the future or worrying about your loved ones, the prescription is the same: bring yourself back to the present moment, as the event hasn't happened yet. Since the event hasn't taken place, the best thing to do is affirm the outcome you want to have happen and focus on that, instead of worrying about what might happen. Most people tend to live in the past or future in their minds, but all that actually exists is the present moment. All you have is this breath. This moment. Now.

REFLECTIONS FROM MY JOURNEY

I grew up with a mother who was a "worry wart" or "nervous Nellie." She grew up with a mother who was a worry wart, and perhaps my great grandmother was also a worry wart. In her book, *Mother–Daughter Wisdom*, Dr. Christianne Northrup writes that we are the culmination of the seven generations that have gone before us. Since I am adopted, I am not sure if worry is a natural, inborn trait and tendency of mine or a behaviour I learned in the environment I grew up in. Nevertheless, I have worked extremely hard to banish worry from my mind. Am I 100% perfect at it? No! Do I have increased awareness about when I fall into this tendency? Yes! By practising the Seven Rs, I fall into this tendency less and less now. That is my hope for you as well.

Step 4: Resolve to repeat

You have to continually interrupt negative thought patterns if you want to have a different experience. Resolve to repeat Steps 1 to 3 until you have retrained yourself and are no longer living unconsciously in your mind. When we are unconscious, it contributes to the experience of depression, anxiety, disordered eating/eating disorders and mania. Ultimately, it is part of the human condition to live unconsciously, but we can break this cycle with awareness.

Resolve to do this process again and again. Why? Because you are human, and it is human nature to get stuck in problematic thinking patterns from time to time. Don't be harsh on yourself. Don't say to yourself "Oh, jeez, here I am, stuck again" in a negative way when you notice you are stuck. Rather, congratulate yourself for noticing. This leads to the road of release.

Step 5: Reaffirm/rephrase

A key step is to rephrase whatever the "negative" thought was that you recognized was keeping you stuck. I typically write in my journal or repeat out loud the opposite thought. For example, if I was thinking "I am not very good at drawing," then the rephrase could be something like, "I let my creativity flow in wonderful ways."

REFLECTIONS FROM MY JOURNEY

It took me many years to be open to the idea that my thoughts affect my mental health and the reality of my world. As I mentioned, if you had imparted Louise Hay's mantra "Change your thoughts, change your life" on me when I was deeply depressed, I probably would have rolled my eyes at you and walked out of the room. When people would say things like this to me, I felt like they were blaming me for being depressed, like it was in my locus of control and all I had to do was "think positive" and I would magically be cured.

Now that I am on the other side of depression, and have more awareness and insight into how my mind works, I can absolutely see the relationship between my thoughts, my physiology and how I feel. The challenge for me, when I was depressed, was that it was too big of a leap to go from "I hate myself" to the rephrase of "I love myself." It felt like a lie. For many, affirmations don't come naturally. It has taken me over 35 years to view the cup as half full versus half empty. But you have to start somewhere.

Even though affirmations can seem like putting the cart before the horse when you are depressed, I have learned that this is an important step in retraining your mind. By repeating affirmations that feel uncomfortable and practising this step, they eventually become familiar and part of your new mindset. Initially, affirmations felt unfamiliar to me because I had never been taught to think like that. There are many things in life that don't feel comfortable the first time we try them, but with practice, they become second nature. It is no different when working with your mind.

If you are reading this and are 10/10 depressed, it is important to understand that your judgment and perceptions may be clouded or distorted. However, this is not *you*. This is what depression does *to* you. You *can* change your thoughts. You don't have to believe every thought you have. You have to learn to become objective about your subjective reality. When you are stuck in it, it is difficult to see the cloud of depression in front of your eyes: it's so thick that you become the cloud. It is important to understand that on a soul level, *you* are still there. You are behind the cloud. And that cloud will lift and the sun will appear again in your life. You can learn to manage your mind; you are not at the mercy of it.

If you find that rephrasing is too big a leap for you, then my suggestion is to stay neutral. For example, in my case, it was too big a leap to rephrase "I am unlovable" to "I am lovable." As such, the neutral, unbiased thought "I am" felt more realistic to me. By staying neutral and non-descriptive, we bring awareness to the labels and judgments we use unconsciously every day. With the insight of awareness, you invite change. We have to be careful how we talk to ourselves because we are listening. By refraining from following negative trains of thought, we condition ourselves to adapt and respond more appropriately to life's events.

Many times, our thoughts are sticky, and simply doing the breath work outlined in Step 3 is not enough. If you find yourself ruminating about something, it can be helpful to ask yourself whether you have taken anything personally or made an assumption. If it is the former, your job is to let it go by using the breath. A useful quote to remember by Dr. Wayne

Dyer is, "Other people's opinions of you are none of your business." As a former people pleaser, I had a hard time understanding that quote initially. But over time, I have learned to let other people's opinions of me go and to focus on the only opinion about me that matters: mine.

If you find you are making assumptions about a situation or person, the best thing to do is check in and clarify what you are thinking. It is best to deal with the facts of a situation versus the fictional story you make up in your head, which may not be true.

This step is about getting underneath the problematic thought to uncover a belief—either conscious or subconscious—that may be keeping you stuck. You can resolve to repeat the first few steps of this process, but to get to healing, you have to unravel your beliefs. Often, it is our beliefs that drive our emotional reactions. By looking at what is behind the behaviour, we gain insight into how to move forward. There are many useful tools that can help with this step. One is Byron Katie's four-question inquiry. The other is cognitive behavioural therapy (CBT). Both tools address our beliefs.

There are two types of beliefs: core beliefs and/or shadow beliefs.

Shadow beliefs

The phrase "Whenever you point your finger at someone, there are three fingers pointing back at you" describes the concept of shadow beliefs. Shadow beliefs are parts of ourselves that we don't realize we possess or don't like, love or accept. As defined by Debbie Ford in *The Shadow Effect*, a shadow belief is an unconscious belief that influences our entire lives, tells us what we can and cannot do, and drives our behaviours. It can also hold you back without you even being conscious that this is happening.

For example, if we are triggered by someone or see something we don't like in them, such as someone being manipulative or deceitful, we project that we don't possess those same qualities. However, most of us do. When you judge someone, you need to look under the judgment at the feeling that is there. The judgment is saying more about you—the judger—than about the person being judged. It is something about yourself that you are disowning and distancing yourself from and putting on to someone else. The key is to ask, "What is the feeling that I don't want to feel?" The people in our lives reflect parts of ourselves that we aren't willing to look at. These represent our shadow beliefs.

Scott Fenstemaker writes about shadow beliefs in his blog (people triggers.wordpress.com):

Shadow Beliefs are the exaggerated or irrational beliefs about one-self about which one is not fully conscious and that can perpetuate unwanted behaviour. That "shadow" part of the term is Jungian and signifies the unconscious and un-dealt-with nature of the belief. A lot of neurotic or otherwise unwanted behaviours are linked to irrational beliefs about ourselves and our abilities.... This can produce varying degrees of unexpected behaviour, ranging from despair to self-sabotage to compulsiveness to social awkwardness.

REFLECTIONS FROM MY JOURNEY

I have had to work through many of my own shadow beliefs, or "unconscious commitments," in the process of writing this book. There have been many fears keeping me stuck in sharing my story. The teaching, counselling and guidance of Nancy Levin, author of *Jump! And Your Life Will Appear: An Inch-by-Inch Guide to Making a Major Change*, has helped me tremendously. The "jump" I wanted to make was to be able to stand in my bipolar truth with no fear. But I needed to heal my heart first.

At one point in the coaching process with Nancy, I came up with the excuse that I needed to wait until my son had graduated from university before I disclosed the truth of my experience living with bipolar disorder. When I shared that with my husband, his response sparked a lightbulb in me. He said, "Well, I think it worked out just fine for Justin Trudeau." For those who may not be familiar with this famous Canadian family, Justin's mother, Margaret Trudeau, also lives with bipolar disorder, and she was married to Pierre Trudeau, a Canadian prime minister whose son Justin is the leader of Canada as I write. This comparison and the guidance from Nancy helped me let go of my fears that my son will be ostracized, ridiculed, shunned or mis-treated because of my illness.

At the end of the day, I believe we all just want to be loved and accepted. That is what I want, not only for myself, but for everyone.

In the coaching I received from Nancy Levin, I learned that one way to uncover shadow beliefs is to look at the choices we make or don't make. Our choices reveal the truth. Every choice we make either serves us or sabotages us. Often, we will make what we think is the easier choice, especially in areas of our lives where we feel the most challenged. For me, I felt it was easier to stay in a well-paying job than to risk rejection while looking for another one or to start my life over in pursuit of my mental well-being and happiness. For someone who wants to lose 20 pounds, it can feel easier to stay on the couch than go to the gym. These "easy choices" are, in reality, not easy at all. Furthermore, they are actually harder because they lead to the destruction of what we say we really want. Why would we be willing to destroy our own dreams? What would drive us to rob ourselves of what we want?

When I reflect on my experiences and struggles, they all eventually boil down to needing to feel security and love. What keeps us from this are unconscious commitments, or shadow beliefs. The problem is we don't remember forming these beliefs, as they are often established in childhood in response to some event or circumstance. A clue to whether there is an unconscious commitment operating behind the scenes in your life is to pay attention when you say you want something but don't follow through with action. This is a red light indicating that there may be a shadow belief that needs to be unveiled before you can move in the direction of your desires and dreams.

By understanding that we create what we are most committed to, we can uncover what is blocking us. Go easy on yourself here. This process is not about blaming or criticizing yourself for being in the same place yet again. We need to be gentle with ourselves because we have made a promise to ourselves in the past—that we would never be hurt, alone or unsafe—that we simply don't remember. We have continued to fulfill this past promise to ourselves up until this day. It is through a process of inquiry, understanding, compassion and awareness that you will realize that you no longer need to keep this promise. You aren't in childhood anymore. These inconsistencies or patterns that keep showing up in your life are reminders that you can either listen to or ignore. I urge you to listen. By listening, you will be able to choose a new, empowering conscious commitment that can guide you in the direction you want to go.

By looking at the emotions that underlie our behaviours, we can get a glimpse into our shadow beliefs. The "how" of what we do shows us what we are committed to. On the flip side, it shows us where we are being held back. Debbie Ford suggests starting with the following three steps.

Step 1: Journal to get in touch with your pain and emotions. I frequently say, "You can't heal it if you don't reveal it."

Step 2: Once you are feeling that pain or emotion, try to connect it to your past to uncover where that pattern of pain began. This step is not about going into detail about the story around a past trauma and reliving it. Instead, the goal is to identify what beliefs you have derived as a result of the event. It is about tapping in to the emotion to reveal the unconscious commitment you have made.

Step 3: Embark on a healing ritual that will help you surrender that pain once and for all. A healing ritual that allows you to be an active participant in love and compassion for yourself is ideal. My healing rituals are journalling, the Seven Rs of working with problematic thoughts and breaking the thought–emotion cycle, meditation, gratitude, nature walks and prayer.

It is important to be patient and kind with yourself. Recognize that shadow beliefs cause you to make the same mistakes over and over again. By reflecting on these patterns in your life, you will be able to unveil the shadow beliefs that may be sabotaging your well-being.

Core beliefs

Core beliefs are like shadow beliefs in that they may be unconscious, but often we have awareness of them. They are beliefs that are typically created in childhood and now run the operating systems of our lives. They drive our behaviours and can serve to propel us forward in our lives or keep us stuck. It is important to assess the validity of our core beliefs. Are they really true? How do they serve us? Many core beliefs may remain fixed in our minds if they develop from a traumatic experience. From a young age, core beliefs help us make sense of our world, and we often fail to evaluate whether they are still useful to us as adults.

Often, identifying these beliefs is enough to understand a recurring problem. But core beliefs don't always reveal the entire story. Identifying core beliefs we have about others and the world can give us a greater understanding of why we might find a situation distressing.

An exercise in uncovering core beliefs comes from working with the Seven Rs of problematic thoughts and breaking the thought–emotion cycle. Often, what lies behind the thoughts that we recognize as "stinking thinking" or emotional reactions are core beliefs. For example, at a young age, I translated being adopted to mean that I wasn't wanted or lovable, and this correlated with emotional patterns of feeling abandoned, overlooked and unwanted. Often, the emotional patterning and beliefs that form in childhood manifest as depression, addiction, anxiety and other mental emotional problems in adulthood. Other common core beliefs are:

- I am not worthy of happiness.
- I deserve to be punished.
- I am stupid.
- I am bad.
- I am worthless.
- I am a loser.
- I don't deserve good things.
- I am a failure.
- I am weak.
- I am not enough.
- I don't matter.
- I am boring.
- I am crazy and unstable.
- I can't be fixed.
- I always hurt people.
- I always hurt myself.
- I have no hope.
- I am a mistake.
- I am helpless.
- I am ugly.
- I am shameful.
- I am inadequate.
- I am unlikeable.

This is not an exhaustive list. It only shows a sample of the many possible core beliefs that could exist within you. There can be more than one core belief operating behind the scenes. Also, we can have core beliefs about others or the world, such as people are mean or the world is not safe. Negative beliefs about the world are more common if you have had a traumatic experience, such as growing up with an alcoholic or drug-addicted parent, sexual abuse or economic hardship. Children growing up in these environments are vulnerable to forming negative core beliefs about the world and others; however, core beliefs can develop at any age.

One way to identify core beliefs is to look for recurring themes as you work with Step 1 of the Seven Rs. Some clues are:

1.   Assumptions that start with "If . . . then . . ."
2.   Sentences that start with "I should."

3. Phrases that start with "I am _____" or "Others are _____" or "The world is _____."

Another exercise to uncover core beliefs comes from cognitive behavioural therapy; it is called the downward arrow technique. In this exercise, you pick a thought that you recognize as "sticky" for you and ask, "What does this say or mean about me?" You may have to continue to ask yourself the question "What does this say or mean about me?" more times than outlined on the next page, or you may arrive at a core belief after asking the question a few times. End the exercise when you arrive at an absolute statement about yourself.

Cognitive behavioural therapy teaches that the next step to working with core beliefs is to gather evidence that doesn't support the belief. You have to build a new belief highway in the opposite direction. This is extremely important, as we may have adopted many core beliefs that simply aren't true or applicable.

Look for evidence that contradicts your belief. In the above example, take note of loving acts or gestures no matter how small or insignificant. Examples include a stranger smiling at you, your pet wagging their tail when you come home, or a friend cooking you dinner. Learn to see love. It also helps to express gratitude and return love when you recognize it. There is some truth to the cliché, "Smile and the world smiles with you."

What I teach patients is to rephrase the negative core belief or thought by replacing it with a more positive or affirming belief that is the opposite. In this example, the opposite statement is, "I am likeable." If we want to feel differently, we need to think differently. When you are depressed, it can be a big leap from disliking to liking yourself. If this is the case, then bring awareness to the descriptive labels you are using. Instead of saying, "I am likeable" or "I am unlikeable," stay in the neutral zone, with, "I am." This exercise gives valuable insight into the adjectives we use and the strong influence of our judging mind. It opens our eyes to the yin and yang elements of our beliefs.

⚷ *As you go about your day, bring awareness to the descriptive labels you use that are mostly negative or positive. If they are mostly negative, see if you can remain neutral instead. In your* **Moving Beyond** *journal, reflect on this exercise and what you learned about yourself.*

Another way to challenge the absolute statement that results from the downward arrow technique is with Byron Katie's four-question inquiry.

DOWNWARD ARROW TECHNIQUE
....

Thought from the Seven Rs exercise:

What does this say or mean about me?
↓

What does this say or mean about me?
↓

What does this say or mean about me?
↓

What does this say or mean about me?
↓

Note: For core beliefs about others, ask, "What does this say or mean about other people?" For core beliefs about the world, ask, "What does this say or mean about the world?"

Here is an example of using the downward arrow technique:

Thought from the Seven Rs exercise: I called Joanne to see if she wants to go to a movie and she hasn't returned my call.
↓

What does this say or mean about me?
Joanne doesn't like me.
↓

What does this say or mean about me?
I am a terrible person; no one wants to be around me.
↓

What does this say or mean about me?
I am unlikeable.

Byron Katie is a self-help psychology author and speaker. She is best known for her teachings on The Work, a method of self-inquiry aimed at working with and through difficult thoughts that lead to difficult emotions. The essence of The Work is to use four questions when faced with any difficult thought:

1. Is it true?
2. Can you absolutely know that it's true?
3. How do you react, what happens, when you believe that thought?
4. Who would you be without the thought?

Here is another way to ask these questions:

1. Is it true?
2. Can you know, 100% without any doubt, that it is true?
3. How do you feel when you think that thought?
4. How do you feel when you don't think that thought?
5. Which thought are you going to think?

I find this process stops negative thinking in its tracks. Most thoughts, when examined under the lens of truth, end up dissolving. Essentially, you are asking if your thoughts are a true reflection of the reality around you or a product of something else—some filter or conditioning program in your mind.

At one point, I had the opportunity to see Byron Katie speak, and she said that we all judge. Immediately, I had the thought "What is she talking about? I am not judgmental. I don't judge people." At the break, I was stunned when I caught myself thinking as someone walked by, "I would never dress like that," which was followed by "Those shoes don't go with that outfit," which was followed by "Oh my gosh, look at me judging!!" I realized that this was a shadow side that I had not acknowledged.

In my opinion, Byron Katie's work is similar to CBT in that it decomposes and challenges thoughts to expose the truth. CBT is based on the theory that much of how we feel is determined by what we think and the thoughts we have. By correcting faulty thinking patterns, we can change the way we view events and positively affect our emotional state.

With CBT, thoughts are examined by writing down what automatically arises in response to a situation, then determining which is the "hot" thought—the thought that has the most impact, emotional charge, or trigger for you. You then come up with evidence that supports that thought, as well as evidence that does not support it. Ultimately, a more balanced thought is created that reflects the reality of the situation. Often, the problem with depression is that it clouds our judgment; we remain focused on what is wrong and fail to acknowledge what we might be doing right. We become blind to the strengths, gifts or positive contributions that we bring to situations.

Categories of distorted automatic thoughts

When I first did CBT as a patient, I found the term "automatic thoughts" confusing because while they were automatic, I was not aware of them. As I continued to journal and build awareness of what was going on inside my head, it became apparent that most of my thoughts were not in support of me. There are also many categories of automatic thoughts that we all have in common, as shown below.

DISTORTED AUTOMATIC THOUGHT	SOLUTION
Mind reading: You assume you know what people think without having sufficient evidence. "He thinks I'm a loser."	Remember the Four Agreements (see page 65)—in particular, the agreement about making assumptions. When we are mind reading, we are making assumptions. Instead of coming up with a story in your head that is completely off base, check in and get the facts so you can stay in the reality of the present moment.
Fortune telling: You predict the future negatively. Things will get worse or there is danger ahead. "I'll fail that exam" or "I won't get the job" or "I won't get better."	Stay in the present and don't make assumptions. Recognize that the future hasn't happened yet. Because of that, it is best to focus your attention on an outcome that you want to have happen, not on all the negative, fear-based outcomes. You can be prepared, if you like, for worst-case scenarios, but it is best to envision a positive outcome and direct your thoughts toward that.

DISTORTED AUTOMATIC THOUGHT	SOLUTION
Discounting positives: You claim that the positive things you or others do are trivial. "That's what spouses are supposed to do, so it doesn't count when she's nice to me" or "Those successes were easy, so they don't matter."	Develop self-compassion by acknowledging your successes.
Negative filtering: You focus almost exclusively on the negatives and seldom notice the positives. "Look at all the people who don't like me."	Gather evidence that contradicts negative filters. Start with gratitude.
Over-generalizing: You perceive a global pattern of negatives based on a single incident. "This generally happens to me. I seem to fail at a lot of things."	Take generalizations through Byron Katie's four-question inquiry; stay neutral and/or use the opposite affirmation.
Dichotomous thinking: You view events or people in all-or-nothing terms. "I get rejected by everyone" or "It was a complete waste of time."	Break down dichotomous thinking with Byron Katie's four-question inquiry; stay neutral and/or use the opposite affirmation.
Shoulds: You interpret events in terms of how things should be rather than focusing on what is. "I should do well. If I don't, then I'm a failure."	In Gestalt psychotherapy, "should" is a swear word. The goal is to stop "shoulding all over yourself." This word often comes from someone else's belief or opinion, and leaves you stuck in guilt and feeling like a victim. Replace "should" with your own belief and rephrase to: I will, I won't, or I need.

DISTORTED AUTOMATIC THOUGHT	SOLUTION
Personalizing: You attribute a disproportionate amount of blame to yourself for negative events, and fail to see that certain events are also caused by others. "The marriage ended because I failed."	Practise the Four Agreements; don't take things personally; remember that "other people's opinions of you are none of your business"; make the Seven Rs of working with problematic thoughts a daily habit.
Blaming: You focus on the other person as the *source* of your negative feelings, and refuse to take responsibility for changing yourself. "She's to blame for the way I feel now" or "My parents cause all my problems."	Remember that every time you point the finger at someone, there are three fingers pointing back at you. Ask the question "What does this say about me?" Take responsibility for what you bring to your encounters with others.
Unfair comparisons: You interpret events in terms of standards that are unrealistic. For example, you focus primarily on others who do better than you and find yourself inferior. "She's more successful than I am" or "Others did better than me on the test."	Often our struggles lie in the gap between the comparisons we make and our expectations that differ from the reality we experience. When we learn to let go of expectations and recognize that when we compare, we are stuck in our egoic mind, we can find lasting peace and joy.
Regret orientation: You focus on the idea that you could have done better in the past, rather than on what you can do better now. "I could have had a better job if I had tried" or "I shouldn't have said that."	When we focus on the past, we are not living in the present. All we can do about the past is change our relationship to it in the present by learning to accept the lessons, honour the struggle and be kind to ourselves in the process. The idea of soul contracts is also helpful with shifting out of regret orientations because you become open to the idea that everything happens for a reason (see Chapter 20).

DISTORTED AUTOMATIC THOUGHT	SOLUTION
What if? You keep asking a series of questions about "what if" something happens, and you fail to be satisfied with any of the answers. "Yeah, but what if I get anxious?" or "What if I can't catch my breath?"	Stay in the present moment and recognize that the future hasn't happened yet. Therefore, it is best to focus your attention on an outcome that you want—not on negative, fear-based outcomes. Prepare for worst-case scenarios if you like, but envision a positive outcome and direct your thoughts toward that.
Emotional reasoning: You let your feelings guide your interpretation of reality. "I feel depressed; therefore, my marriage is not working out."	The solution to emotional reasoning is to practise the Seven Rs of working with problematic thoughts and breaking the thought–emotion cycle. Also, emotional reasoning relates to making assumptions. Therefore, check in with the emotion to determine if the thought patterning is true. Get the facts.
Judgment focus: You view yourself, others, and events in terms of evaluations as good/bad or superior/ inferior, rather than simply describing, accepting or understanding. You measure yourself and others according to arbitrary standards, and find that you and others fall short. You focus on your own and others' judgments. "I didn't perform well in college" or "If I take up tennis, I won't do well" or "Look how successful she is. I'm not successful."	Mastering Byron Katie's four-question inquiry is extremely helpful with shifting out of judgment. It is also helpful to bring awareness of the descriptive labels we use and to try to stay neutral, i.e., "I am" vs. "I am not successful."

Step 6: Reflect

This step is about learning. With each episode of depression, anxiety, mania or binge eating that I have had, I have reflected on what happened by asking the following questions:

1. How did I get sick?
2. Was there something I missed?
3. Did I stop exercising?
4. Did I stop eating properly?
5. Did I stop taking my supplements/medications?
6. How have I been sleeping?
7. Is there something that I want to say to someone that I am not saying?
8. Was I under stress?
9. Did something change in my environment—a move, a new job, the loss of a relationship?
10. Did I stop being mindful?
11. Did I take something personally?
12. Have I made an assumption?

By looking backwards, we can prevent future relapses in our mental health. I have stumbled many times, and it has taken several attempts to get on solid emotional ground. I have put in the work, read many self-help books, taken the courses, made huge life changes, eliminated toxic relationships, and set boundaries—all in support of my health and well-being. I wouldn't be where I am today without the important step of reflection.

Step 7: Reward

This is really a step that my husband added. He said, "If you are going to do all that hard work, you might want to reward yourself." This step speaks to the love and compassion part of the diagram on page 74. You have to treat yourself kindly to love yourself. I find it helpful to remember that you are going to be with yourself longer than anyone else is going to be with you—longer than your parents, siblings, cousins, partner, children, friends, co-workers. So, it is vitally important in building your self-esteem that you get the relationship right with yourself first before seeking love from another. By rewarding yourself with a kind gesture or simple life pleasure—whether curling up with a good book, getting a massage, having nice warm bath, watching a movie, buying yourself flowers or going for a walk in the forest—treating yourself with love, kindness and compassion will allow it to flow from you to others.

In my practice, I ask patients to work with these seven steps and breathing exercises whenever they recognize their thoughts as negative. But there are also several other times throughout the day that I ask patients to pause with their breath. The idea behind this is that the more you engage in deep, rhythmic diaphragmatic breathing, the more you shift your physiological state to one of calmness instead of stress and anxiety. Remember that when we do this, our nervous system shifts to a parasympathetic state. The times that I encourage everyone to take a few deep breaths are: when you wake up in the morning, before eating, after going to the bathroom, whenever you are in a line-up, when driving (with your hands remaining on the wheel, of course!) and before bed. The more times throughout the day that you can reset yourself, the less chance anxiety has of getting a grasp on you.

For many, learning to manage the "monkey mind" is the key to transforming fear. Fear is an especially loud monkey, sounding the alarm incessantly, pointing out all the things we should be wary of and everything that could go wrong. Buddha showed his students how to meditate to tame the monkeys in their minds. It's useless to fight with the monkeys or try to banish them from your mind because, as we all know, that which you resist persists. Instead, Buddha said, if you will spend some time each day in quiet meditation—simply calming your mind by focusing on your breathing or a simple mantra—you will, over time, tame the monkeys. They will grow more peaceful if you lovingly bring them into submission with a consistent practice of meditation.

I've found that the Buddha was right. Meditation is a wonderful way to quiet the voices of fear, anxiety, worry and other negative emotions.

*To master these steps, your homework is to write down thoughts that you recognize as "sticky" or "hot," as well as the reframes of those thoughts. Keep your **Moving Beyond** journal with you as you go about your day, and practise the Seven Rs daily, including the breathing exercises.*

REFLECTIONS FROM MY JOURNEY
....

In my experience, engaging the monkeys in gentle conversation can sometimes calm them down. I'll give you an example. In my life, fear seems to be
an especially noisy monkey, especially around being self-employed and having
to rely on myself versus the security of a corporation for my livelihood. With
the recessions of recent years and the crumbling of pension plans and job
losses, I know more and more that security is an illusion. As the years go by,
Fear Monkey shows up less often, but when he does, he's always very intense.
So, I take a little time out to talk to him.

"What's the worst that can happen?" I ask him.

"You'll go broke," Fear Monkey replies.

"OK, what will happen if I go broke?" I ask.

"You'll lose your home," the monkey answers.

"OK, will anybody die if I lose my home?"

"Hmmm, no, I guess not."

"Oh, well, it's just a house. I suppose there are other places to live, right?"

"Uh, yes, I guess so."

"OK, then, can we live with it if we lose the house?"

"Yes, we can live with it," he concludes.

And that usually does it. By the end of the conversation, Fear Monkey
is still there, but he's calmed down. And I can get back to work, running my
practice and living my life.

Pay attention to how your monkeys act, listen to them and get to know
them, especially the Fear Monkey. Take time to practise the Seven Rs of
working with problematic thoughts and breaking the thought–emotion
cycle on a regular basis. Learn how to change the conversations in your
head. Practise kind, loving, compassionate self-talk and see how it can
transform your fears and your life.

The Seven Rs of working with problematic thoughts and breaking the
thought–emotion cycle are the foundational framework needed to build
the pathway to mental freedom. If you stick with this and continue to
practise it daily, you will change your default programming. The levels
of mental anguish you experience will decrease. There may still be trials

or tribulations in your life or things to address, get over or get out of, but you now have the tools to deal with the storms of your life from a place of calm-centred peace versus panic-riddled anxiety.

I believe one of the greatest travesties of the 21st century is the rising rate of mental illness and the disengaged approach to life that so many people seem to have. Too many don't care whether they will live to see another day. There is a silent epidemic going on with respect to mental illness, and the medical community and media have been talking about it for several years now. It is time to turn the conversation into action, into change, into freedom for those who are suffering.

(19)

Emotions—Behave and React in the World

"Ultimately, the goal is to learn to respond from a place of emotional calm, like a still lake, versus reacting with disruptive emotional waves, like a lake in stormy weather."

DR. CHRIS

I OFTEN FIND THAT patients have a hard time connecting to their emotions. It is important that you know that you are not alone if this is an area that you struggle with too. Know that it is common to be at a loss for words when it comes to describing your emotions.

The question I ask patients that they find the hardest to answer is "What is the main emotion you experience throughout the day?" Take a moment to answer that question before reading on. If you need help determining the answer, consult the emotional regulation chart on the next page.

*In your **Moving Beyond** journal, use the emotional regulation chart to write a list of emotions that resonate with you, and write down a list of emotions that you are disconnected from. Write about how you are navigating the emotional tides of your life. Are you drowning in discomfort, or swimming with success?*

There are a few key points that I want to highlight about this chart:

1. All emotions are normal.
2. Emotions have an energetic quality to them. As such, they are to be released. They are not meant to be stuffed, suppressed, choked back,

UPWARD SPIRAL

Freedom

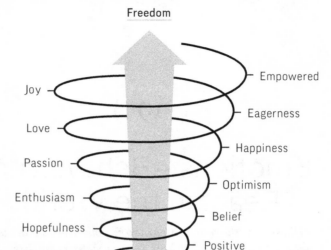

Joy

Love

Passion

Enthusiasm

Hopefulness

Contentment

Empowered

Eagerness

Happiness

Optimism

Belief

Positive
Expectations

- - - - - - - - - - - - - - - Boredom - - - - - - - - - - - - - - -

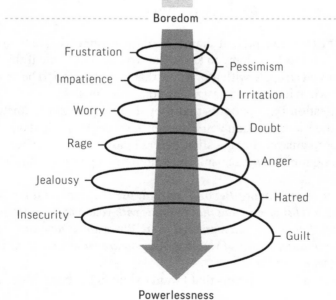

Frustration

Impatience

Worry

Rage

Jealousy

Insecurity

Pessimism

Irritation

Doubt

Anger

Hatred

Guilt

Powerlessness

DOWNWARD SPIRAL

EMOTION CHART

SOURCE: Hicks, Esther and Jerry. *Ask and It Is Given: Learning to Manifest Your Desires*. Hay House, 2004.

held in, pushed down, stifled or not unexpressed. If you do any of the foregoing (or anything but express them), it is very important that you do the exercises in this chapter. Your health depends on it.

3. Emotions can be managed and regulated once they are expressed and understood.
4. There is no need to be afraid of your emotions.

Many people with mental health issues have a hard time accepting themselves. By using the Seven Rs of working with problematic thoughts and breaking the thought–emotion cycle, I have garnered awareness about my emotions and feelings.

REFLECTIONS FROM MY JOURNEY

In the past, if you had asked me if I am an angry person, I would have said no. Anger was not an emotion that I was connected or in touch with. I think that was partly because I spent an entire decade battling with depression and thoughts of suicide. Underlying that depression was a lack of self-love and compassion. I found it hard to love myself when I was operating on the faulty core belief that I was unlovable and unwanted. The other part about anger was that I did not like feeling out of control emotionally. I also had a deep fear of going manic. As a result, I felt I had to keep a lid on my emotions. I couldn't get too angry, excited or happy for fear of what someone else might think or how I would be judged.

While it is important to learn to embrace our emotions, I believe understanding our level of sensitivity is also necessary. There are some people who are an empathic or emotionally sensitive person (ESP), others who are a highly sensitive person (HSP), and some who are both. These terms often get lumped together, but they have different meanings. Most experts agree that all "empaths" are highly sensitive, but not all highly sensitive people are empaths. Here's how to distinguish between them:

An ESP is a person who can feel the emotions or physical symptoms of others even if they themselves are not going through the same situation or event. It is estimated that approximately 2% to 3% of the population are ESPs.

"HSP" is a term used to describe a person who has high sensory awareness and often feels extremely emotional or in-tune with their surroundings. It is estimated that approximately 15% to 20% of the population is highly sensitive.

To put it simply, ESPs pick up on energy, whereas HSPs pick up on sensory stimuli.

The two books on this topic that I recommend are:

- *The Emotionally Sensitive Person: Finding Peace When Your Emotions Overwhelm You* by Karyn D. Hall
- *The Highly Sensitive Person* by Elaine Aron

About being emotionally sensitive, Karyn Hall writes:

When you're emotionally sensitive, you experience emotions more intensely than others. Your feelings of love, joy, happiness, anger, sorrow, and fear are stronger than average. If you aren't able to manage your emotions, you struggle every day to cope. You sometimes don't trust yourself because you can't predict how you'll react in different situations. Too often, your emotions get the best of you, and you act on them in ways that aren't helpful in making your life better—sometimes adding more anguish and trouble to your life.

Emotionally sensitive people have a deeply sensitive perspective of the world, such as being connected to animals and nature more than most. They are generally attuned to the emotions of others and can exhibit both excessive tolerance and intolerance. Most have rejection sensitivity and can easily perceive rejection in everyday situations, such as an email or text that isn't returned. They're intuitive thinkers and often can't verbalize how they know what they know. They have difficulty making decisions, a strong sense of justice, and a fluid sense of identity.

In terms of being highly sensitive, Elaine Aron defined a population of people having "increased sensitivity to stimulation" and who "are more aware of subtleties and process information in a deeper, more reflective way." After reading her book *The Highly Sensitive Person*, I realized that I am highly sensitive. I have since embraced my sensitivity as a gift versus a personality flaw. I encourage you to take the "Are You Highly Sensitive?" quiz on the next page to see if you are highly sensitive.

ARE YOU HIGHLY SENSITIVE?

....

Answer each question according to the way you feel. Answer true if at least somewhat true for you. Answer false if it is not very true or not at all true for you.

1. I seem to be aware of subtleties in my environment.   T_____ F_____

2. Other people's moods affect me.   T_____ F_____

3. I tend to be very sensitive to pain.   T_____ F_____

4. I find myself needing to withdraw during busy days, into bed or into a darkened room or any place where I can have some privacy and relief from stimulation.   T_____ F_____

5. I am particularly sensitive to the effects of caffeine.   T_____ F_____

6. I am easily overwhelmed by things like bright lights, strong smells, coarse fabrics or sirens close by.   T_____ F_____

7. I have a rich, complex inner life.   T_____ F_____

8. I am made uncomfortable by loud noises.   T_____ F_____

9. I am deeply moved by the arts or music.   T_____ F_____

10. I am conscientious.   T_____ F_____

11. I startle easily.   T_____ F_____

12. I get rattled when I have a lot to do in a short amount of time.   T_____ F_____

13. When people are uncomfortable in a physical environment, I tend to know what needs to be done to make it more comfortable (like changing the lighting or the seating).   T_____ F_____

14. I am annoyed when people try to get me to do too many things at once.   T_____ F_____

15. I try hard to avoid making mistakes or forgetting things.   T_____ F_____

16. I make a point to avoid violent movies and TV shows.   T_____ F_____

17. I become unpleasantly aroused when a lot is going on around me.
    T_____ F_____

18. Being very hungry creates a strong reaction in me, disrupting my concentration or mood.   T_____ F_____

19. Changes in my life shake me up.   T_____ F_____

20. I notice and enjoy delicate or fine scents, tastes and sounds, works of art.   T_____ F_____

21. I make it a high priority to arrange my life to avoid upsetting or overwhelming situations.   T_____ F_____

22. When I must compete or be observed while performing a task, I become so nervous or shaky that I do much worse than I would otherwise.   T_____ F_____

23. When I was a child, my parents or teachers seemed to see me as sensitive or shy.   T_____ F_____

SCORING YOURSELF

If you answered true to 12 or more of the questions, you are probably highly sensitive.

But frankly, no psychological test is so accurate that you should base your life on it. If only one or two of the questions are true for you, but they are extremely true, you might also be justified in calling yourself highly sensitive.

SOURCE: Aron, Elaine. *The Highly Sensitive Person: How to Thrive When the World Overwhelms You.* Broadway Books, 1996. All rights reserved. Reprinted by arrangement with Kensington Publishing Corp. www.kensingtonbooks.com

....

Most of the bumps in my relationships have been due to the messy combination of sensitivity, a lack of self-worth, an unconscious need to test people's love, and the tendency to make assumptions—a dangerous mix, let me tell you! Over the years, through all the bumps and bruises, I have learned to interpret my emotions so I can positively influence the outcome. I have learned to navigate the emotional waters of my life by understanding boundaries and practising the Four Agreements.

Boundary work

The key to understanding your emotional reactivity is to understand the concept of boundaries. Boundary setting is challenging for most of us because we are taught to put others' needs, wants and desires ahead of our own. The attachment we feel to putting others first is difficult to break free from. As such, pleasing becomes the way we seek and obtain love. The good news is that every time you say yes to setting a new boundary, you are saying yes to more freedom.

In order to set a new boundary, you have to take your own needs into consideration and prioritize them. It means being conscious about choosing yourself over another person and not reacting or responding to someone else's demands, requests, drama, needs or crisis. Setting new boundaries will allow you to act from a place of intention and truth. Maintaining the new boundary goes hand-in-hand with setting the new boundary.

This discussion about choosing yourself over another gets controversial because we are so used to putting other people's needs ahead of our own. This is especially true for women. Many find it is a huge shift to put their own needs first. So, I want to be clear that I am *not* saying to discount the needs of others or neglect your responsibilities. Instead, I want you to gain insight into the ways you default when a request is made of you. Do you automatically respond "Yes," and regret your answer a minute later? Are you afraid to disappoint anyone, and subsequently that fear takes precedence over the boundary you are trying to maintain? Ultimately, boundary setting is a call to self-inquiry about what you really want and desire.

As you begin to set new boundaries, you can feel off-balance and maybe even a little scared. When you start to operate from the place of what you want, it can feel like you are speaking a new language for the first time. At times, it will feel challenging to set a new boundary because you are so used to taking care of everyone else. Remember, there is no need to pretend that you are a superhero. The goal is to start rescuing yourself instead of everybody else. An important reason to commit to this process of setting new boundaries is because when you don't, you end up demonstrating and reinforcing the beliefs that run your inner dialogue, such as:

- "I am not enough."
- "I am not lovable."
- "The needs and opinions of others are more important than my own."
- "If I disagree with someone or ask for what I want, I will end up alone and unloved."

As discussed in Chapter 18, these are examples of beliefs that run in the backgrounds of our minds and contribute to our fears about setting boundaries. If you dig deeper, you might find that you have adopted these beliefs from someone else. These other people have taken up residence inside your head. Wherever these opinions come from, it is your job to disengage and find your own voice. As you do, you will undoubtedly experience natural reactions that inhibit your progress and keep you stuck. Change is hard for most of us. Remember that there are no rewards when you rest in resistance. You will find yourself coming up with excuses for why you can't set boundaries and worrying about what will happen if you do.

Pay attention to the excuses you use and how you might justify why you can't set a boundary. A good place to begin is to start saying no when you typically would have said yes. Or you can respond by saying, "Thank you for asking me. Can I get back to you?" This gives you the time and space you need to really check in with yourself about where your yes is coming from. Determining where your yes is coming from is a major component of boundary work. What is the driving force, intention and motivation that is the basis for your yes? There is a cascade effect to setting boundaries. Setting the first one will help you develop the courage to set another.

🔑 *Take a moment to visualize yourself saying no when you know you need to take care of yourself. Imagine meeting your own needs first. Imagine giving yourself what you need and satisfying your own internal desires instead of searching for that outside of yourself.*

Setting boundaries

The first question to ask yourself is "Do I know when my boundary has been crossed?" For the benefit of those who answer no, the answer is that your boundary is crossed whenever you say yes to a request when you really mean no. Have you ever been in the position where someone asks you to do something, and before you take a moment to think about whether you actually want to fulfill the request, you automatically blurt out "Yes" without thinking? Then, the minute they walk away, you find yourself wishing you had said no. That is a subtle, yet powerful, example of a boundary crossing. The goal is to make sure that when we say yes to any request, we mean it. To do this, we must change our immediate response from "Yes" to "Can I get back to you?" Then it is important to take some time to journal or reflect on the request. Do you want to do it? If not, then a suitable response is "Thank you for asking me; however, I am unable to help now." If you can offer another solution, then great! But don't feel obligated, as it is not your problem to solve.

Most of us stretch ourselves too thin because we fill our time with too many activities, requests, errands and obligations, and don't allow ourselves enough time to get things done. Then we feel stressed, which leads to irritability and frustration. Remember: when you say yes, you want it to be a true "yes."

🔑 *In your **Moving Beyond** journal, reflect on whether you ever say yes when you really mean no. Can you think of a recent example from your life when you said yes and later wished you had said no?*

Another example of understanding boundaries comes from our emotions. At times, our boundary is crossed when we have a negative emotional reaction. This can be as subtle as saying to yourself, "Hmmm, I wonder what she meant by that comment," or as obvious as bursting into tears at an offhand remark, or getting frustrated with your child because they are running late for school. There is usually a palpable sigh of relief in the room when I share my own struggles and frustrations with my depressed patients who are parents. It helps them come out of the shame closet when they know they are not alone. What is important is learning how to stop the shame game and manage our emotions effectively. Learning to set boundaries has been a key step in regaining my mental health. I was so attached to keeping others happy that it superseded my own needs. I admittedly suffered from the disease to please.

Here are the steps that have helped me tremendously:

Step 1: Boundary crossing recognition
Steps 2 to 5: Emotional regulation
Step 6: Getting professional help

To navigate the emotional waves of our lives, we need to follow boundary road signs:

Step 1: Recognize that your boundary has been crossed. Your boundary may be crossed whenever you find yourself in emotional waters that are uncomfortable, or you find yourself saying yes to requests when you really mean no. Remember that the level of discomfort is not as important as having awareness that you are feeling uncomfortable emotionally.

Step 2: Find out whose issue it is. With boundary crossings that relate to emotional reactions, the question to ask yourself is "Whose shit is this and whose diaper is it in?" Essentially, you are trying to determine whether you have something unresolved in you, they have something unresolved in them, or you both have unresolved issues.

If you recognize that it's *your* shit in *your* diaper, then your job is to do the work to resolve whatever emotional issue you might have that is smouldering in you. Ask yourself: "Have I taken something personally?" If yes, your job is to let it go by doing the breath work outlined in Step 3 of the Seven Rs of working with problematic thoughts (see Chapter 18). Remember, a key concept is that "Other people's opinions of you are none of your business." Pause and read that quote again slowly: "Other people's opinions of you are none of your business." Many people suffer from the "disease to please," including myself. As a recovering people pleaser, I can say that letting go of other people's opinions of me has been the medicine I needed. What is most important is not what others think of you, but what *you* think of you—not in a narcissistic way, but in a supportive, considerate, compassionate and loving way.

If you have not taken something personally, then ask yourself: "Have I made an assumption?" If yes, then you need to stay in the present moment with your breath until you can get factual answers about your assumption(s). We always want to deal with hard facts, not the stories we make up in our heads with our "monkey minds."

If you haven't made an assumption, the next step is to see if you can identify a core belief underlying the emotion. If yes, rephrase and repeat Step 3 of the Seven Rs of working with problematic thoughts. If no, bring awareness to your thoughts and write them down in your journal. Review what you have written and identify a thought that seems to be a trigger for you. Challenge that thought with the four-question inquiry of The Work by Byron Katie: 1) Is it true? 2) Can you absolutely know that it's true? 3) How do you react when you believe that thought? and 4) Who would you be without the thought?

If you are still feeling emotionally stuck, or the emotional wave has not subsided or calmed down, then I suggest making an appointment with your naturopathic doctor or counsellor.

☛ *In your **Moving Beyond** journal, write about a time when your boundary was crossed. How did you resolve it?*

Try these simple exercises for uncovering boundary crossings that relate to shadow beliefs:

Exercise 1: For one week, whenever you find yourself overreacting to another person's behaviour, ask yourself: "What traits in that person am I trying to disown in *myself*?"

Exercise 2: Make a list of the advice you give others and ask yourself if the advice is appropriate for your own life. Many people teach what they need to learn themselves.

☛ *For the next week, if you find yourself triggered or irritated by another person's behaviour, answer the following question in your **Moving Beyond** journal: What qualities in that person are you not acknowledging in yourself?*

REFLECTIONS FROM MY JOURNEY

When my son was three years old, I noticed that I was getting very frustrated and that my level of irritation was out of proportion to the situation. I found this emotionally exhausting and did not like the type of parent I was in those moments. I also didn't like the emotional hangover I would have if I lost my temper: shame, blame, guilt, disappointment in myself and beating myself up in my head with negative thoughts. I sought support from my naturopathic doctor, a counsellor and many self-help books.

This is how learning to manage my emotions after my boundary had been crossed looked for me. The incident refers to times when my son isn't listening to me in any given situation (such as getting ready for school, eating dinner, doing chores, getting off screens, getting ready for bed). Note: The emotional rating scale I am using is from 1 to 10, with 10 being the worst.

Incident 1: Lose my temper with no warning or awareness that I am going to lose my temper. Intensity rating: 20/10.

Incident 2: Recognize I am getting irritated, yet am unable to communicate what I am feeling before losing my temper. Intensity rating: 10/10.

Incident 3: Recognize I am getting frustrated; am unable to communicate what I am feeling, but leave the room to do breath work as outlined in Step 3 of the Seven Rs. End up punching the pillow instead while out of my child's sight and earshot. Intensity rating before leaving room: 9/10; intensity rating after punching the pillow: 3/10.

Incident 4: Recognize I am stressed, use my voice and say, "I am feeling really stressed right now" in a not-so-calm tone. Leave the room, punch the pillow, pick up my journal and start writing while doing breath work. Intensity rating before leaving room: 9/10; intensity rating after journalling: 1/10.

Incident 5: Recognize the wave of irritation as it rises in me. Calmly say, "I am feeling irritated right now because I don't feel you are listening to me. If you don't do x by the time I count to five, then you will have to go to your room [or some other consequence].One... two... three... four... four and a half..." Like magic, he responds. Intensity rating before counting: 3/10; intensity rating after counting: 0/10.

The point of this example is to illustrate that this is a process that takes time. With the right tools, level of awareness, self-compassion and understanding, you can learn to manage your emotions and boundaries. Granted, it may take longer if you have serious anger management issues, but you have nothing but time and nothing to lose by putting these suggestions into practice.

In the midst of anger, it can feel like it is the other person who has wronged you. Often, however, anger is a clue that there is something going on with you that has nothing to do with them. It is often a response to your own judgments, the failed satisfaction of your own expectations, or your failed attempts to gain control of your subconscious response to fear. To establish and maintain peaceful relationships with other people, surrender your beliefs by using Byron Katie's four-question inquiry. Learn to suspend judgments of others. of who they are and who they are not. What you have to gain is peace, calm, patience and serenity. Ultimately, the goal is to learn to respond to your life from a place of emotional calm.

O⤚ *In your **Moving Beyond** journal, write about when you recently had an emotional outburst. What was going on? Did you make an assumption? Had you taken something personally?*

I learned to work with my emotions by practising the Seven Rs of working with problematic thoughts and breaking the thought–emotion cycle, as well as using all the boundary steps outlined on page 245.

In this chapter, I have entered the thought–emotion cycle from a different vantage point. Instead of focusing on the thoughts, as in Chapter 18, here you shift your focus to the sensations of irritation, frustration, stress, anger, disappointment, pain or whatever emotion is rising within you. Awareness of the emotional wave is the key. You also need to bring an element of compassion to yourself as you learn this process. As discussed in Chapter 8, the road to recovery is not always linear. It can be a few steps forward and one step back. Overall, the trajectory is forward, and we end up in a healthier place as we learn to manage our thoughts and emotions over time.

It requires patience, figuring out what the lessons are, learning or getting the lessons, and making mistakes to test whether we have truly learned the lessons. But at any point in time, you will see you are making forward progress even if it feels like you aren't.

It has been said that first you get the lesson like a tiny pebble hitting you on the side of the head, then a bigger rock, then a large boulder. In some cases, perhaps the entire mountain has to come crumbling down for you to get the lesson. Hopefully, you learn the lesson after two or three knocks to the head versus a major life catastrophe. Sadly, many people have to hit rock bottom (addictions are one example) before they are ready to make the changes they need.

Another reason you may experience repeated bouts of depression or anxiety—especially when you really thought you were *over* it—is that these continued experiences are allowing you to heal a shadow side or an emotion on another level. In homeopathy, we use the "onion analogy": humans are like onions, and as you peel away the layers, you get closer to the essence. It does not mean you are a failure for not getting the lesson. It means you are in the university of life and still earning your PhD. As you learn to manage your emotions, it is important to remember that things that come up remind you of you and your presence. It can be that there are many layers to uncover. When I experience what I perceive to be a setback, I remind myself that everything happens for a reason. This is based on the idea of soul contracts, which I explain in Chapter 20.

REFLECTIONS FROM MY JOURNEY

Have you ever had an "upset" with someone? Perhaps there is someone in your life who is not talking to you, or vice versa. Many patients mention these situations to me, saying their families are "dysfunctional." What most of my patients don't know is that I have had the same experience with my family and friends. I have been struggling with this for many years: what to do, how to fix it, how to let go. I have spent countless dollars and hours in counselling, and filled many journals, in an effort to resolve these conflicts. I have come to understand that the lessons for me are:

1. The importance of letting go
2. The recognition that other people's opinions of me are none of my business
3. The understanding that transformation happens when we learn to love and accept ourselves
4. The belief that I am good enough and worthy of love, just as I am

A few years ago, I had two larger boulders hit me on the side of the head. The first was regarding an acquaintance on a trip we took together. A few weeks before we were supposed to leave, I recognized a large rock coming at me (that I was trying to ignore) when I found myself thinking, "It would be better if I shortened my trip or cancelled it all together." Did I listen to this message or trust my inner voice? Of course not. I rationalized it away with my ego by saying, "C'mon, you've already paid for your accommodations. Your flights are booked. How will you get your money back? How will you explain that you don't want to go anymore?" Suffice it to say that I did not enjoy myself at all on this trip and ended up wishing that I hadn't gone.

It also ended in a parting of ways with my acquaintance, as I couldn't speak my truth about how I was feeling about the trip, the situation I was in, or my stress levels. On the one hand, I am okay with this. But on the other hand, I have a hard time when I think people don't like me. I seem to give my own opinion of other people less weight than their opinion of me. I seem to disregard my belief that a relationship is no longer a fit for me when I perceive that the other person doesn't like me. In my highly sensitive mind, it is not okay for someone not to like me. I can tell you that this belief has caused me much angst, heartache, energy and upset over the years, as I would go to the ends of the Earth (or sacrifice or suppress my own thoughts and feelings) to save a relationship. I have had many sleepless nights pondering why person X does not like me, or why person Z has not returned my call or email.

That summer, I had another boulder hit me from out of the blue, land on my chest and crush my heart. This was much more difficult than the experience mentioned above, as it involved a family member. Many hurtful things were said to me, and it was a reminder to me to be careful about the words you choose, for they can cut like a sword. In fact, what word do you see when you write "words" with no spaces between them?

wordswordswordswordswordswords

It spells swords! Believe me, what was said cut like a knife right into the deepest part of my soul. To give you an idea, one statement involved a comment about me having a mental illness, and how this family member was "sick and tired of catering to you and your mental illness."

This highlighted to me that there are still many people out there who are not accepting of mental illness and very judgmental. I've often thought that if I had Parkinson's, multiple sclerosis or cancer, people would be more understanding, supportive and accepting. But because my challenges are on the interior, with anxiety, social phobia, depression, an eating disorder and bipolar disorder, people just don't get it. It has become my life's passion and purpose to break these barriers down and crusade for compassion, insight and understanding for those diagnosed with mental illnesses. I have been equally devoted to my own healing, as I grow into my soul recovery and accept responsibility for what I bring to situations. I am also extremely grateful for the people who have stuck by me—whether they understand me or not—like my husband, mother, father, aunt, cousins and many dear friends. I know they love me, and while I used to want them to "get it," I have come to accept that they don't need to. They just need to stand by in love. By doing so, they have showed me how to love myself. Isn't that what it is all about?

In my situation, it is a matter of life and death at times, as I have been affected by depression and plagued by suicidal thoughts. The difference in past years for me in not acting on those thoughts has been the flicker of light shining through the cracks of my broken heart. This light reminds me I have worth despite the judgment of those who have cast me aside for whatever reason. I am still learning to accept the lessons of letting go of the past and other people's opinions. I can tell you that it has freed up time for me, as I no longer spend countless hours writing in my journal or repeatedly analyzing what has happened in my mind. I just breathe in, bring myself back to this moment, this gift in time, and exhale all the self-critical thoughts that I have of others and myself. Slowly, one breath at a time, healing is taking place for me. My wish is it takes place for you too.

This lesson in letting go from Robert Holden's book *Be Happy* is helpful:

> Letting go: Suffering is a decision not to let go of the past yet. Happiness is a decision to step into the present now. And being present is what helps you to **let go of what is not happening now**. You may have had an unhappy childhood, but that is not happening now. You may have experienced a romantic heartbreak, but that is not happening now. You may have had a bitter disappointment in your career, but that is not happening now.
>
> Letting yourself be happy is not a denial that suffering ever happened, and it is certainly not an attempt to dishonour any old pain. Letting yourself be happy is, however, a signal of intent to be free of more suffering. By choosing happiness, you invite healing. By saying "Yes" to happiness, you invite grace. By being open to happiness, you discover you have a deeper compassion for yourself than even you realized. Letting yourself be happy can be translated as **I have suffered, and I want to be free; I feel pain, and I choose joy; I feel fear, and I ask for help; I feel angry, and I am open to forgiveness; I feel sad, and I call upon compassion; I feel lost, and I welcome grace.**
>
> Until you let yourself be happy, you make an idol of your suffering, which prevents you from seeing the true depth and beauty of your

original nature. One of the mantras of my work is "**Pain runs deep but joy runs deeper.**" As you let yourself be happy, you realize that pain and suffering belong to the ego, but true healing and joy belong to your original nature. In other words, you realize that although you have experienced pain, you are not your pain, and that although you may continue to experience suffering, you are not your suffering. **Happiness is giving up all resistance to letting go.**

On a positive note, just two hours after the above-mentioned incident, I was reunited with my favourite aunt from childhood. Due to family and life circumstances, I had not seen her for 11 years. The tears of joy and the loving embrace when I saw her washed away all the pain I had experienced in the hours before.

Rumi said, "Do not look outside yourself and seek love, look within to see all the walls you have built between it and your heart." Ask yourself where you have put a wall in your heart to protect it from being hurt. To break down these walls, breathe in love and, with the exhalation, let love flow or radiate outward unconditionally to your family, friends, co-workers and those you may have a grievance with. I decided to share my experiences as I know that having an "upset" with someone is a common theme in many people's lives. My intention is for this to be helpful to you, so you, too, can get to the place of acceptance, understanding, forgiveness and, finally, letting go.

🔑 *In your **Moving Beyond** journal, write about whether you have put a wall up in your heart to protect it from being hurt.*

It is important to continually ask yourself where you are living in your head. If it is the past or the future, you need to return to the present moment with the guidance of your breath. There is nothing you can do about the past. It is over. Done. Complete. Finished. To leave it in the past, you must accept what has happened, let go of any associated negative emotions (such as bitterness, resentment, disappointment), and forgive.

If you find you are living in the future, then you also need to get back to the present moment, especially if the thoughts you have about the future are founded in worry. Remember that worrying, fretting and distressing yourself over situations has a negative impact on your physiology and contributes to anxiety and depression. Since the future hasn't happened yet, affirm the outcome you want to have happen and spend time visualizing that outcome unfolding. Use the Seven Rs of working with problematic thoughts to guide you in this process.

By working with your emotions and boundaries, and redirecting yourself to the present moment, you will create a permanent shift in your emotional experiences for the betterment of your health.

(20)

Spirituality, Love and Forgiveness

"Remember, you are going to be with you the longest.
It is vital you get the relationship right with yourself
first before seeking love from another."

DR. CHRIS

THINK IT IS important to start this chapter off with a disclaimer: There is a difference between religion and spirituality, and for the purposes of this discussion—and in recognition that there are many religions in the world— I choose to honour and accept them all. For me, what matters is that you are on a loving spiritual path that promotes peace, compassion, acceptance, understanding and respect for humanity. It is not my place to judge which road you choose to take. I have investigated many paths, and I feel they all lead me to the place of healing the heart. For me, spirituality and healing speak to the state of your heart and soul, and that is what I am concerned about. The path you take to get there is secondary, in my opinion.

In this book, I've discussed the "Western" or "scientific" view that mental illness is caused by a biochemical imbalance in the brain, and the corresponding idea that you can treat it by giving the body what it needs—for example, pharmaceuticals that aim to balance neurotransmitters or orthomolecular therapies that provide the correct form of essential nutrients to support the neurotransmitters. In my practice, I have seen this with every patient I treat who has an imbalance in the mental realm; there is no denying the physical and causal connection between neurotransmitters and one's mood state. However, I wanted to share something that might be a little "out there" with you about one of my views about depression and mental illness.

My "out there" view is that mental illness is a way by which our spirit is trying to get our attention because some aspect of our lives (such as school, work or a relationship) is not moving in concert with our spirit or divine plan. That is, maybe we are moving west and our spirit is trying to take us north. By looking at ourselves and taking the time to be silent, talk to others and open up about what we are feeling, we can address the underlying root of depression, anxiety, addiction, bipolar disorder, and other problems that can lie in the spiritual realm. This excerpt from the *Journal of Naturopathic Medicine* highlights the importance of the spiritual aspect of healing:

> The human being is not simply a physical entity. We have minds, we think. We have emotions, we feel and we translate these feelings into meaning. We are spiritual beings.... Causes of disease manifest in four groups or levels: spiritual, mental, emotional and physical. Of these four aspects, the spirit is the centre; the next layer is the mental aspect of the person, then the emotions and the outermost layer is the physical. If there is a distortion on the spiritual level, it will create distortion through the system, like ripples from a stone thrown into a pond.

It is my personal belief that a connection to a spirit, whatever your chosen practice is, is critical and vital to healing yourself and the current state of the planet. I define spirituality as believing in a power greater than yourself. Until my time is up, I won't know the answer to what happens to my soul. For many, the term "soul" or "spirit" is intangible or esoteric. I define your "soul" or "spirit" as your life energy.

When I studied anatomy, we dissected cadavers. The difference between you and a cadaver is life flow. In traditional Chinese medicine, this is referred to as "qi" (pronounced "chi"), or life energy. In this chapter, I will share with you some of my experiences and beliefs that I hope you will find comfort in and resonance with.

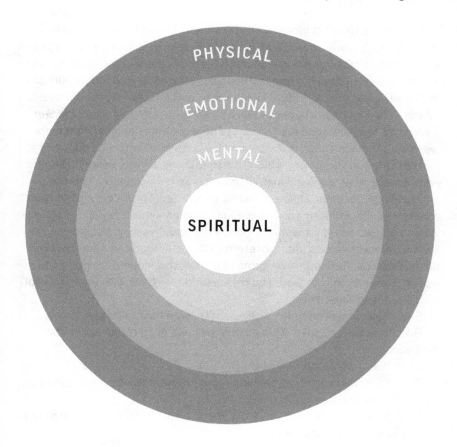

REFLECTIONS FROM MY JOURNEY

As I mentioned before, my recovery from kidney failure was viewed as a miracle by my nephrologist, given the amount of poison I had consumed. I am open to the idea that it was a miracle, as I had so many people praying for me to make a complete physical recovery. I remember when I was recovering in the ICU, one of my friends asked me if I had seen "white lights" and if I was "sent back." As I was still in a state of recovery and hadn't had time to process what had happened, I just shook my head and the conversation moved on from there.

Now, more than 20 years later, the answer I have for why that suicide attempt didn't work when I think it should have is based on the concept of "soul contracts." Basically, if I succumb to suicide in this lifetime, then my soul will not evolve spiritually. I first learned about the concept of soul contracts in Colin Tipping's book *Radical Forgiveness*, and it is also illustrated beautifully in a children's book by Neale Walsch called *The Little Soul and the Sun*. I have come to understand the concept of soul contracts to mean that before we inhabit the human form, our soul makes a contract with God about what our next life will be about—what our experiences will be, what challenges we will have to overcome, what we have come here to learn, who our parents, siblings, partners, children, and so on will be. (Think of "God" or "god" as whatever or whoever you believe in personally—male, female or other.) When we leave the spirit world to inhabit the body, we forget about the contract we made with God until we return to the spirit world as a soul upon our death. Basically, the lessons we come to learn in this lifetime are agreed to in a soul conversation with God. The conversation we have with God as a soul might be along these lines:

Soul: "God, in this lifetime I really want to learn how to forgive."

God: "Are you certain? This means you will go through some painful experiences."

Soul: "Yes, I am certain. I am ready!"

God: "I don't know. It may be hard—you may have to endure abuse, rape, death, trauma and betrayal."

Soul: "I am okay with that, as I trust in you, God. I really want to learn how to forgive on the deepest level."

God: "So it will be."

This concept of soul contracts offers an explanation for the phrase "God doesn't give you more than you can handle." While I have outlined one suicide attempt in this book, there have been other attempts and much too much energy on my part spent contemplating suicide. What shifts me from contemplation is recognizing that suicidal thoughts are the ultimate example of "stinking thinking" and being unkind to myself. By practising the Seven Rs of working with problematic thoughts and breaking the thought–emotion cycle, I can get outside of my head, which gives me a reprieve from these negative thought patterns. By shifting to a place of curious wonder about where these thoughts come from, not attaching to them, and recognizing that in that instance I am being unkind to myself, I no longer ignite suicidal thoughts with fear or a deep disdain for myself.

But before I learned how to do that, it was a single belief—that if I succumb to suicide in this lifetime, my soul will not evolve or graduate and I
must endure this lesson over again—that has helped me stay here with you
on the planet.

My soul has come here to learn how to love myself, how to love others,
and how to live out a full life, and it is not my job to take my life. I believe that I
probably did not survive a suicide attempt in a past life, and that if I die in this
life by suicide, then I may have to repeat this "grade" in soul school the next
time around. For me, it is not about how much money I make, how successful
I am or how decorated an athlete I was. It is about surviving mental illness
and moving beyond the labels into love and acceptance of myself and others.

Remember, we agree to the challenges and difficult times and we are
preparing to do something that we have chosen to do in this lifetime. It is like
you are in boot camp until the moment you are ready to compete. We have
all chosen to be here and to go through lessons in this lifetime. The size of
the lesson doesn't matter. When you come out the other side, that is when
you have learned.

Love for yourself

Ultimately, it is our feelings about ourselves and how we treat ourselves
that are critical to our mental health and well-being. I ask every patient
how much they love themselves on a scale of 1 to 10, and it is rare for me
to get a response over five. The most common response I get is "Now,
that is a tough question to answer." A few patients have responded with
a negative number. This saddens me to the core of my being. It breaks my
heart to hear someone speak so unkindly of themselves, yet I, too, would
once have given a similar response. It is important to look into another
person's eyes with heartfelt caring and loving intent. My response to my
patients is "When I look in your eyes, I only see love and I do not see
anything not to love." But it is one thing for me to say this and another
for patients to embody and accept this statement.

If you talked to your best friend the way you talk to yourself, would
they accept it? When I pose this question to my patients, not once have
I received a reply of "Yes." Many who struggle with mental wellness are

hiding this conversation that they are having with themselves and living in shame.

This is the work we need to set about doing: accepting and loving ourselves. You are a gift to the world—a unique creation—and you are worthy of your own love and acceptance. Recognize that. Feel that. Embody that. And give that love to yourself. Then give it others.

Not acknowledging your strengths, gifts, accomplishments and achievements is a way of putting yourself down and keeping yourself small. The world wants to see your light. As Marianne Williamson writes in *A Return to Love*: "Our deepest fear is not that we are inadequate. Our deepest fear is that we are powerful beyond measure." If we learn to move through fear, self-doubt and criticism and embrace love, then our true self can shine through.

Getting started

When you don't love yourself, how do you start? A great place is mirror work. I learned this exercise from Louise Hay's book *You Can Heal Your Life*. Start by looking at yourself in the mirror—connecting with your eyes—and saying, "I love you." If emotions come up, be with them. It is important to pay attention to how you do this exercise—from not doing it at all, to how long you are able to look at yourself, to the thoughts that might arise as you do it.

It's important to do this exercise frequently. Just as brushing our teeth is a daily hygiene habit, we need to make loving ourselves a daily hygiene habit as well. One of the reasons this is so difficult is that, as children, many of us aren't taught we have worth. Depending on the core beliefs we formed in childhood, the "love for oneself" muscle may be weak and need a lot of strengthening. If you were told as a young child not to be conceited or boastful or, even worse, endured abuse at the hands of another, then extra effort might be required to build your self-esteem. We have to give to ourselves first and look inside ourselves for the answers that we are looking for.

Since you are going to be with you longer than anyone is going to be with you, it is important to get that relationship right before seeking love from another. The famous line from the movie *Jerry McGuire*—"You complete me"—couldn't be more wrong. You should complete you, not someone else.

🔑 *Make loving yourself a daily habit by doing the mirror exercise. In your **Moving Beyond** journal, write a list of things you love about yourself. Program three of these qualities into your phone as a reminder and reflect on them a few times a day. Or write them on sticky notes and put them around your house, in your car or on your desk as reminders to appreciate these loving qualities that you possess.*

Another way to love yourself is to note what you appreciate about yourself. Many patients say they don't feel they have any good qualities or strengths to acknowledge. I ask them to complete an online survey that assesses character strengths (the VIA Character Strengths questionnaire—see www.viacharacter.org). The test was co-created by Dr. Martin Seligman (commonly known as the "father of positive psychology" and author of *Authentic Happiness* and *Flourish*) and Dr. Christopher Peterson, author of *A Primer in Positive Psychology*. The VIA Character Strengths survey provides useful information that can help you understand your positive strengths. Most personality tests include negative or neutral traits, but this survey focuses on your best qualities.

🔑 *Take the VIA Character Strength Survey. In your **Moving Beyond** journal, write about an experience in which you utilized one of your strengths.*

REFLECTIONS FROM MY JOURNEY

When I was first diagnosed with bipolar disorder, my psychiatrist recommended not to disclose my mental health condition to anyone in the workplace. He felt it was still very misunderstood, that a huge stigma existed, and that I would feel any repercussions more keenly due to working in the conservative banking industry. He did not want anything to be used against me or to jeopardize my possibilities for future promotions. We all know that business politics can be cutthroat.

On the one hand, I agreed with his advice, especially the part about jeopardizing my career. The unfortunate aspect was that wearing the mask of "everything is okay on the outside, but I am dying on the inside" only served to perpetuate the shame and stigma, not break down the walls of misjudgment that surround mental illness. I felt I had to hide this part of myself because it was not acceptable to others. When I experienced dark days of depression, it was very hard to reach out and ask for help because of the mask I constantly put on for work, and because the voice in my head was constantly berating me with abusive thoughts of how useless I was.

The slow process of learning to love and accept myself started in 1994, after my suicide attempt, when I read Marianne Williamson's book *A Return to Love*. I have subsequently read many books on self-help and healing. For me, the biggest spiritual lessons along the way have been identifying my soul contracts, acknowledging, accepting and reframing my shadow and core beliefs, loving myself, learning to trust my inner voice, letting go, and forgiving.

Learning to trust your inner voice

In spiritual circles, many speak about "the voice." We all have a voice in our head that keeps talking and talking, and many of us are completely absorbed by it. This is the voice that tells you why you aren't good enough, that keeps you fearful or keeps you in analysis mode so you never end up making a decision. That is the wrong voice to listen to. When I suggest you learn to trust your voice, I am referring to your inner voice: the voice of truth that is always trying to get you to listen. There are many expressions for the idea of an inner voice: intuition, inner guide, sixth sense, gut feeling, soul, spirit, heart, voice of God, etc. I will use them interchangeably in this chapter. This is the voice that is trying to get you to live your purpose.

The important questions are: Can you hear it? And if yes, do you listen to it? Learning to trust your inner voice is an integral part of healing. Intuitively, your body knows what to do to repair and self-heal. The problem for too many of us is that we don't trust it. Instead, we remain in doubt, fear, depression, anxiety and indecision. Lack of confidence, indecision and self-doubt are all symptoms of depression that cloud our judgment and make it difficult to trust our intuition.

REFLECTIONS FROM MY JOURNEY

When you are guided by your inner voice, the next steps in your path become clear. For example, I initially asked to take a sabbatical from my corporate career and planned to use that time to determine my next steps. But my request was denied. So, I was forced to decide: continue at my job or resign. Amid fear and self-doubt, I resigned. I set out to go back to school to become a naturopathic doctor, but I lost my confidence and felt like it was going to take too long. The road to becoming a naturopathic doctor was frightening compared with other options that seemed easier, but were full of roadblocks.

I ended up trusting my inner voice that said to become a naturopathic doctor, even though I was scared to do so. I had spent months reflecting on the question "If money didn't matter, what would you being doing with your life?" and the answer that consistently revealed itself to me in tiny whispers was to become a naturopathic doctor so that I could help people heal from the same mental health challenges that I have overcome—anxiety, depression, eating disorders, bipolar disorder type 1, addiction and so on—using natural therapies and orthomolecular medicine. Immediately, my next thought was "You can't do that! You're 33 years old, at the height of your career—you'd be a fool to start over now." But in the end, I didn't let the voice of fear stop me.

I now know that my inner voice is the only one to listen to. I no longer feel paralyzed by angst when making decisions. I may not understand why I'm following the voice, but I don't argue with it. What you have to gain from learning to trust your inner voice is peace of mind, inner strength and joy. It also protects you from danger. Just as animals use their senses to protect themselves from danger— for example, fleeing to higher ground in the event of a tsunami—we have our own inner intelligence. It is that voice that says "Don't accept that drink" or that feeling inside that says "Go left instead of right." Your intuition is a built-in security guard.

To learn to trust your inner voice, follow these steps:

1. Be silent

I often say to patients that it is difficult to hear the voice of God if you are always talking. While prayer is a useful tool for many, it is still thought-based. To hear your inner voice, silence is required. Developing a regular breathing practice sharpens your awareness skills. It is through silence, stillness and an aware presence that your inner voice can be heard. The more you ppractise the Seven Rs of working with problematic thoughts and breaking the thought–emotion cycle, the more clearly you'll hear your inner voice.

2. Reconnect with your body

Our bodies are always talking to us. That is why descriptive terms to describe your intuition include things like "gut instinct" and "spidey sense." I can literally feel tension around my stomach and heart when my intuition is trying to get my attention. A simple exercise to help you trust your inner voice (versus the voice of fear) is to start having a conversation with your heart. For example, in any given situation, you can pay attention to the response your body gives you when you ask Yes or No to a question you have or a decision you are trying to make. If you notice a warmth or softening in your body, then the answer is Yes. If you feel a contraction, heaviness or closing, then the answer is No. The key is to figure out how your body communicates with you. Different people have different ways of tuning in to their inner voices.

3. Listen to messages from the heart

A common concern is differentiating between the voice of the heart and the voice of the mind. If you aren't used to tuning in to your gut feeling and trusting it, you might doubt its message at first. It would be nice if we could just call 1-800-DOUBT for assistance. Since that hotline doesn't exist, we end up calling someone who knows us for help and advice, often a parent, sibling, best friend, colleague or therapist. By talking to someone who knows us, we hope to get clear answers. The key is to learn to trust yourself for the answers versus searching outside of yourself.

When it comes to "matters of the heart," the answer resides in you. It requires listening. Start by having a conversation with your heart around simple decisions, such as: "Tonight, would you like brown rice or quinoa for dinner?" Slowly work your way up with these small decisions so that you can build your confidence when it comes to making bigger life decisions. I encourage you to check in with your heart for the small decisions you make every day, such as what to wear, which route to take when driving, what to order if you are eating out, what to watch on TV or what to cook for dinner. For any question, consult your heart and it will give you an answer. Learn to listen. Most importantly, learn to trust the answer.

It is one thing to differentiate your inner voice from the many other thoughts coming from your mind, another to trust it, and still another to act. The more you listen and act, the easier it gets. Learning to act despite fear is what is necessary. A book that helped me with this is *Feel the Fear and Do It Anyway* by Susan Jeffers. The goal isn't to eliminate fear, but to trust your heart in the face of fear and understand that fear is part of the process.

HOW TO LISTEN TO YOUR INTUITION
....

It took me a long time to listen to my intuition. I hope I can make this a little easier for you by suggesting these tips:

1. Observe and discern between the physical body sensations associated with a yes or no response to your questions.
2. Practise listening to your inner voice with small daily decisions.
3. Act.

A practical exercise you can do to build your intuition is to leave the house with no plans. You can step out for an hour or make it a whole-day adventure. Either way, tune in to your feelings and allow them to guide you about where to go. The key is to not have a pre-set agenda—just enjoy every step you take and follow where your intuition guides you. Be completely present and notice what happens and where you go. If you like, you can set an intention before you leave and see if what transpires.

  ⚷ *Do the above exercise and write about your experience in your **Moving Beyond** journal.*

Heart exercise

Learning to trust my intuition has been a work in progress for me. I can tell you that every single time I didn't, I ended up admitting that my gut instinct had been right in the first place.

The heart exercise, developed my Mastin Kipp, has been helpful for me, and I use it with patients to initiate a connection with one's intuition. You can either have a friend read the questions below or you can close your eyes and say them to yourself.

Place your hands on your heart and pay attention to how you feel around your heart. Say out loud, "Heart, show me where you are" and notice if there is a sensation, feeling, colour or word that comes up. If there is a sensation, breathe into it and stay focused on it as you ask the next questions. Repeat the question out loud and verbalize any answers that come up for you:

1. Heart, will you ever lie to me? Yes or no?
2. Heart, will you always tell me the truth? Yes or no?
3. Heart, have I always followed you? Yes or no? If the answer is no, ask your heart how it feels when it recalls that you haven't always followed it. For example, if the response is "sad," the next question is: Heart, why do I feel sad right now? The response may be something like "Because you've betrayed me" or "You don't listen to me."
4. Heart, can you forgive me for not always following you? Yes or no?
5. Heart, can you help me forgive myself for not always following you? Yes or no?
6. Heart, is it possible that you are God, grace or my intuition dwelling within me? Yes or no?

You can have a conversation about anything. The heart answers in very simple terms: yes, no, stop, go. The mind is complicated, but the heart is simple. It will always give you the right answer. If you start doubting or feeling fear, ask, "Heart, is that you speaking, or is it my mind?" as the mind wants a say.

This self-inquiry is free and available to you always. When you do it, you will find that your anxiety calms and events feel less stressful. You are silencing the mind with this exercise.

Let's be clear about the role of the mind: you need your mind to help you figure out *how* to do what the heart wants. If it is the other way around and you use your mind to lead the way, you may stay stuck or run into obstacles. I find this quote by Joseph Campbell helpful to remember: "The heart must usher the mind into the zone of revelation." I interpret this to mean that we must lead our lives from a heart-centred place. The heart will give you answers that will freak out the mind. Ultimately, part of the spiritual journey is learning to trust the heart's response and follow through even if it scares us.

Forgiving and letting go

For many, forgiveness is a tough step. It is natural to want to curl up, protect, blame, defend or retreat when you perceive that you have been wronged. I know that for me, it has become one of my life missions to truly forgive those who have hurt me or whom I have harmed. Understanding the concept of soul contracts helps us move into forgiveness because everything that happens in our lives is for our growth, learning and evolution. Easier said than done, I know.

As Buddha said, "Holding on to anger is like drinking poison and expecting the other person to die." In other words, anger, bitterness and resentment only hurt you. A useful barometer for me in terms of where I am in forgiveness with someone else is how I feel when I think of that person. I often say to myself if I am ruminating about a past transgression: "I doubt so-and-so is giving *you* any thought or energy, so when are you going to let it go and move on?"

HOMEWORK

. . . .

Some important questions to reflect on by writing in your *Moving Beyond* journal are:

1. Who in my life do I need to forgive?
2. Is there anyone I am harbouring resentment or ill-will toward, either consciously or subconsciously?
3. Who am I slightly angry at or bitter toward in my heart?
4. How do I get to the place of forgiveness?
5. How do I know when I have truly let something go?

REFLECTIONS FROM MY JOURNEY

I find that the concept of forgiveness comes up most during times of celebration, such as at Christmas. This is a time when emotions can run higher for many reasons: expectations, past hurts or disappointments, pressure to see and do too much, over-indulgence in food and drink.

To this day, I reminisce fondly about our family's Christmas traditions, from our "Charlie Brown" Christmas tree, to setting out the decorations, to me forcing the questions "Who is this Jesus character anyway, and why is He so important?" to the scrumptious Christmas treats and turkey feast, to visiting family.

Even so, starting from my teenage years, I began to notice problems. My parents didn't seem that happy in their relationship. My brother, who is four years older than I, was up to no good with his teenage antics. When he was 19, he went travelling to Australia for an indefinite period; my parents divorced that fall. After that, Christmas was not much fun anymore for me. I felt torn between my parents, I felt obligated to make Christmas a joyous time for my mom, and I wanted everyone to get along. This coincided with the start of my mental health challenges.

A few years ago, I was talking to my mom about our family dynamics, with particular reference to the Christmas season. She shared with me why Christmas was difficult for her. She grew up with an alcoholic father and a mother who had to sneak out of the house to work to feed her children. As a result, my mom looked after her younger brother and did the household chores so her father would not take his anger out on them. It is easy to understand why she has bad memories, and equally understandable that she sought a better experience for her own children.

When her father died in a drunk-driving accident at the age of 50, my mom was finally able to relax a little, knowing the worries about his alcoholism were finally over and she could begin healing on an emotional level. Now, more than 50 years later, she is still healing. As she said to me, "I don't get it. I keep busy, I keep on doing things, and then out of the blue, the feelings just well up inside of me and the tears start flowing. I know where it stems from—my dad, and now your brother."

My response to her was: "Mom, the wound from the memory of your dad is so deep that it cuts to the centre of your being. The reason you keep so busy is to avoid feeling. But the healing is in the feeling. It takes time, sometimes it takes a lifetime, but you only have this one life to live. It is your choice: keep on doing and running, or stop and feel it—all of it. Let the tears flow like a stream, river, fountain, waterfall, ocean or tsunami and allow the healing process to start. Eventually you will feel better and the tears will stop flowing.

"Right now, it is like you have a dam or wall of protection built up inside you from the experience of having an alcoholic parent. You don't have to defend yourself anymore and you can release that pain for good. Visualize all the pain that these two have caused you as a sack of rocks you have been carrying over your shoulder for decades. It is heavy. Now, imagine setting that sack down and walking away, and notice the lightness you can feel in your being when you sigh a deep breath of relief from letting go. Now is the time to let go."

With each year that passes, I continue to reflect on the concept of forgiveness. For many, a part of the healing puzzle includes our capacity to forgive; however, forgiveness is not always easy. This is partly because we may feel that by forgiving someone, we are saying, "That's okay"— that their behaviour or transgression is acceptable. This is not what forgiveness is. By forgiving, you are not condoning the behaviour; you are releasing yourself from the trap of resentment. You are saying, "The way you treated me, or your behaviour, is not necessarily excused; however, I release and forgive you, as well as myself." The Bible advises us to "forgive them for they know not what they do." That is what forgiveness is about. For many, saying "I forgive you" leaves the other person stuck in the energy of blame. If we are to be responsible for our actions and perhaps our contribution to the event, a gentler approach is to say, "I am sorry this happened between us."

It is important to understand that forgiveness is about freeing ourselves, not necessarily the other person. It allows us to heal mentally, emotionally and spiritually. We can expend a lot of energy when we hold someone out of our hearts. Holding a grudge, standing in the energy of hatred and resentment, harms us as much as it does the other person. However, when we let go and forgive those who have hurt us, the energy shifts between us, allowing emotional freedom.

To quote Dr. Christianne Northrup:

Forgiveness moves our energy to the heart area, the fourth chakra. When the body's energy moves there, we don't take our wounds so personally—and we can heal. Forgiveness is the initiation of the heart, and it is very powerful. Scientific studies have shown, for example, that when we think with our hearts by taking a moment to focus on someone or something that we love unconditionally—like a puppy or a young child—the rhythm of our hearts evens out and becomes healthier. Hormone levels change and normalize as well. When people are taught to think with their hearts regularly, they can even reverse heart disease and other stress-related conditions. The electromagnetic field of the heart is 40 times stronger than the electromagnetic field produced by the brain; to me, this means that every cell in our bodies—and in the bodies of those around us—can be positively influenced by the quality of our hearts when they are beating in synchrony with the energy of appreciation.

Dr. Northrup also takes readers through a powerful forgiveness exercise in her book *Women's Bodies, Women's Wisdom*. This exercise has helped me heal the hole in my heart that was caused by unresolved conflict in my relationships. I urge you to practise this exercise as well by recording the message in your own voice and playing it back to yourself after you have spent some time in silent meditation or prayer.

FORGIVENESS MEDITATION BY STEPHEN LEVINE

Close your eyes...

For a moment just reflect on what the word forgiveness might really mean. What is forgiveness?

And now, very gently—no force—just as an experiment in truth—just for a moment—allow the image of someone for whom you have much resentment—someone for whom you have anger and a sense of distance—let them just gently, gently, come into your mind—as an image, as a feeling.

Maybe you feel them at the centre of your chest as fear, as resistance.

However they manifest in your mindbody, just invite them in very gently for this moment—for this experiment.

And in your heart, silently say to them, "I forgive you. I forgive you for whatever you have done in the past that caused me pain, intentionally or unintentionally. However you have caused me pain, I forgive you."

Speak gently to them in your heart with your own words—in your own way.

In your heart, say to them, "I forgive you for whatever you may have done in the past, through your words, through your actions, through your thoughts that cause me pain, intentionally or unintentionally. I forgive you. I forgive you."

Allow... Allow them to be touched... just for a moment at least... by your forgiveness. Allow forgiveness.

It is so painful to hold someone out of your heart. How can you hold on to that pain, that resentment even a moment longer?

Fear, doubt... let it go... and for this moment, touch them with your forgiveness.

"I forgive you."

Now let them go gently, let them leave quietly. Let them go with your blessing.

Now picture someone who has great resentment for you. Feel them maybe in your chest, seeing them in your mind as an image—sense their being. Invite them gently in.

Someone who has resentment, anger—someone who is unforgiving toward you.

Let them into your heart.

And in your heart, say to them, "I ask for your forgiveness, for whatever I may have done in the past that caused you pain, intentionally or unintentionally—through my words, through my actions, through my thoughts. However I caused your pain, I ask your forgiveness. I ask your forgiveness.

Through my anger, my fear, my blindness, my laziness. However I caused you pain intentionally or unintentionally—I ask your forgiveness."

Let it be. Allow that forgiveness in. Allow yourself to be touched by their forgiveness.

If the mind rises up with thoughts of self-indulgence or doubt, just see how profound our mercilessness is with ourselves and be open to the forgiveness.

Allow yourself to be forgiven.

Allow yourself to be forgiven.

However I caused you pain, I ask for your forgiveness. Allow yourself to feel their forgiveness.

Let it be.

Let it be.

And gently… gently… let them go on their way in forgiveness for you—in blessings for you.

And turn to yourself in your own heart and say, "I forgive you" to you.
Whatever tries to block that—the mercilessness and fear.
Let it go.
Let it be touched by your forgiveness and your mercy.
And gently, in your heart, calling yourself by your own first name, say, "I forgive you" to you.
It is so painful to put yourself out of your heart.
Let yourself in. Allow yourself to be touched by this forgiveness.
Let the healing in.
Say, "I forgive you" to you.

Let that forgiveness be extended to the beings all around you.
May all beings forgive themselves.
May they discover joy.
May all beings be freed of suffering.
May all beings be at peace.
May all beings be healed.
May they be at one with their true nature.
May they be free from suffering.
May they be at peace.
Let that loving kindness, that forgiveness, extend to the whole planet—to every level of existence, seen and unseen.
May all beings be freed of sufferings.
May they know the power of forgiveness, of freedom, of peace.
May all beings seen and unseen, at every level of existence, may they know their true being.
May they know their vastness—their infinite peacefulness.
May all beings be free.
May all beings be free.

○⚮ *Take the time to do the forgiveness meditation. Write in your Moving Beyond journal about this experience. Who came forward for you? Where you surprised? Was it who you expected?*

Each time you do this exercise, you will get closer and closer to forgiveness.

Stepping out of blame and conflict

Forgiveness allows you to step out of blame and conflict—which otherwise keep you stuck in a state of fight, flight or freeze—to a place of where you can start to process your emotions and learn to befriend yourself and others. Ultimately, our survival as humans depends on our capacity to cooperate with others, and that includes extending compassion to your own heart. It is possible to allow yourself to purposely and intentionally open your heart.

Usually, when there is conflict in your relationships with others, it means you need to shift an emotion inside of you. When we aren't connecting with others, it is because we aren't connecting with ourselves. To move to a place of healing, we need to pay attention to what is going on internally. The first step in moving to compassion and forgiveness is to come back to your heart, where the emotion resides in you. By directing our focus inward, we can see where we need compassion, attendance and healing. To do this, we have to let go of blame.

To facilitate this process, it can help tremendously to create time in your life for reflective journalling. The gift that journalling, mindfulness and self-compassion brings is it eases our emotions and allows them to be released. When we shine the light of attention on our emotions, the grip starts to loosen and allows a shift in the sense of who we are. We move from being a victim—wronged, angry, hard done by or wounded—to a place of compassionate understanding with oneself. It is this shift in identity that needs to happen. When spiritual leaders talk about how to evolve the collective consciousness, it is really this shift from a place of ego that says, "I'm right, you're wrong"; "I'm good and you're bad"; "Do it this is way, not that way"; or "You're the enemy and I am innocent" to that place where we can tune in to ourselves and be kind, so we can unlock that stuck place inside us. As that begins to unwind, we can communicate with others in a way that moves toward mutual understanding.

Here is a story of a Student talking to a Master that illustrates this point:

Student: "My life is like shattered glass; my soul is tainted with evil. Is there any hope for me?"

Master: "Yes, there is something whereby each broken thing is bound again. And every stain made clean."

Student: "What?"

Master: "Forgiveness."

Student: "Whom do I forgive?"

Master: "Everyone in your life. God. Your neighbour. Especially yourself."

Student: "Well, how is that done?"

Master: "By understanding that no one is to blame. No one."

"There is no one to blame" is the core insight—especially when we accept the idea of soul contracts. Blame will block our ability to be present to the unfolding and processing of our emotions. The Seven Rs of working with problematic thoughts and breaking the thought–emotion cycle can create a ripple effect that is part of the collective healing of ourselves and our Earth.

Given my personal trials and tribulations over the years, there have been loved ones who have also gone through difficult times because of my challenges. I consider my true friends and family members to be the ones who are still by my side despite my hardships, struggles and difficulties. What saddens me to my core is the inability of some individuals to forgive events or actions that have taken place when I was mentally unwell.

If you are struggling in a relationship, see if you can accept that there might be an emotion stuck in you or you may have a shadow belief. Begin to bring an honest, healing presence to what resides in you. Use the Soul vs. Ego chart on the next page to move from your ego into your soul.

SOUL	EGO
Truth	Truth
Conscious	Unconscious
Love	Fear
Surrender	Expectation
Knowledge	Perception/Interpretations
Innocence	Sin/Guilt/Punishment
Faith/Trust	Hope
Empathy	Sympathy
Essence	Form
Joy	Must be Right
Responsibility	Blame
Willing	Trying
Connection to the Divine	Beliefs/Thoughts/Feelings
Joined	Attack/Defence
Constant	Changes
Light	Body
Consciousness of Deserving	Money/Sex
One with God	Separation
One with All	Separation
We are One	We are Separate
Peace	Pleasure/Pain
Eternal	Sickness/Death

Affirmation: I am ready, willing and able to fully accept myself as I am.

🔑 *Write in your **Moving Beyond** journal about someone you might be blaming for a circumstance in your life or with whom you have an "upset." Perhaps there is someone who is not talking to you, or to whom you aren't talking? What emotion might be stuck in you? Use the Emotion Regulation chart (page 238) and the Soul vs. Ego chart as guides to where you might be stuck.*

I feel you have truly forgiven someone if you can see them anew the next time you encounter them. If seeing them doesn't conjure up memories of the old wounds, incidents or acts, then the seeds of forgiveness have been planted, nourished and will continue to flourish. If you can truly feel joy and love when you think of them, and not dig up the hatchet you have buried, then you have forgiven.

Gratitude

If you don't already have a spiritual practice, be open to how you can integrate one into your life. It can be as simple as saying "thank you" every morning. I used to go to bed every night and pray that I would die in my sleep. When I woke up the next morning, I would say to myself, "Oh, God, not another day" and pull the sheets over my head, not wanting to face the world. Now, I go to bed grateful for the day that I have just lived. When I wake up in the morning, I say to myself with a smile, "Thank you, God, for another day."

What a shift. Spiritual practices are as varied as people in the world. The main idea is to take a larger perspective and develop a daily practice of getting in touch with that which is greater than you. If you need a place to start, I recommend starting with gratitude. A useful quote to remember is this one by Master Eckhardt: "If the only prayer you ever say your entire life is thank you, it will be enough."

*In your **Moving Beyond** journal, make it a daily practice to write down three things you are grateful for each day.*

(21)

Common Myths About Mental Illness

"With awareness of faulty beliefs in the present moment,
we can change our future behaviour."

DR. CHRIS

THE PSYCHIATRIC MEDICAL community (and society in general) tends to believe and promote a number of myths about mental health. In fact, many of the false ideas outlined below have been conveyed to me by medical professionals or people in passing before they knew I had bipolar disorder. Since you may have come across these myths as well, or may even be harbouring some of them yourself, I'd like to wrap up this book by debunking them.

Myth #1: If you have a mental illness, you should not have children because it is genetic.

A small component of some mental health disorders may be linked with genetic inheritance. But the much stronger determinant of a person's mental health is learned—temperament, disposition, coping strategies, inner strength—and can be cultivated with mindfulness. In fact, going through something as intense as recovering from mental illness can make a person stronger and more compassionate (and certainly much more aware), and can help a child develop awareness of themselves as they grow.

Myth #2: Your mental health issues will worsen with age.

Your brain can change as you get older; some mental health concerns do progress with age. However, mental health is extremely individual. The changes that occur in one person with age will not necessarily occur in others. With treatment and monitoring, illnesses can stabilize or even go into remission. Also, we now know more about neuroplasticity—your brain's ability to change. You can build new neuronal pathways in your brain, and these can change the course of your mental illness.

Myth #3: It will take six weeks for vitamin, herbal, homeopathic or pharmaceutical medications to work.

Although various medications can sometimes take up to six weeks to take full effect, other benefits begin almost as soon as you start taking them. Often the act of seeking support and beginning treatment with a professional helps a patient gain confidence that they are being well looked after. An often difficult part of mental illness is the despair that things will not get better. Beginning treatment gives hope that can help sustain someone until clinical effects begin to kick in. Also, it does not necessarily take the full six weeks for this to happen. Many people begin to feel some improvement within two or three weeks.

Myth #4: It is hard to come off an antidepressant or psychotropic medication.

This is what I have been told by every psychiatrist I have ever seen except for one: Dr. Abram Hoffer. In order to stop taking antidepressants and other psychotropic medications, you must do two important things. First, believe it is possible. Second, correct any underlying nutritional deficiencies. If you simply stop taking a medication or reduce the dose, you may have trouble because you haven't changed the underlying environment in which your neurotransmitters and hormones are made. It is important to ask your health care provider the right questions. "How do I support the production of neurotransmitters naturally?" Or put another way, "Why am I not making enough serotonin, dopamine or GABA?" Once you build in the correct foundation in conjunction with the medication, it makes for a smoother transition, depending on the medication's half-life. Know that there is another way, and you can come off medications under the supervision of a qualified health care practitioner who understands the importance of nutritional and herbal medicine in conjunction with pharmaceuticals. It does not have to be difficult. You will have to make changes. Be prepared. You've got this! Medications that I have easily come off of using these suggestions include: imipramine (Tofranil), desipramine (Norpramin), lorazepam (Ativan), valproic acid (Epival), carbamazepine (Tegretol), dextroamphetamine (Dexedrine), lamotrigine (Lamictal), fluoxetine (Prozac), sertraline (Zoloft), buproprion (Wellbutrin), olanzapine (Zyprexa), citalopram (Celexa) and lithium carbonate (Lithobid).

Myth #5: You cannot manage mental illness without medication.

This myth is perpetuated by the medical establishment and pharmaceutical industry. It goes hand-in-hand with the myth that vitamins and minerals are ineffective in treating mental disorders. The tragedy of modern medicine is that it is not simply directed by what is best for patients. Politics and economics have encroached their way onto the stage and direct the research, support and finances that lead the philosophy and practice of medicine in certain directions. Often when someone develops a mental illness, particularly depression or anxiety, one of the first people they contact about it is their family doctor. Many doctors believe that depression and anxiety are caused by a chemical imbalance in the brain—low levels of serotonin, to be specific. As such, medications are typically the only solution offered, and what patients typically hear is, "This is all there is." Pharmaceutical medication may be one way to support neurotransmitter formation; supporting biochemical imbalances through nutritional means is another option. The truth, however, is that there is evidence for the effectiveness of other treatment methods, both naturopathic and conventional, especially in combination.

Mental health can be cyclical in nature, but this does not imply the need for constant medication to prevent further episodes. When the root cause of the mental imbalance is treated from its nascence, the symptoms will not reappear. This is achieved through therapy, natural treatments, habit formation and self-care. If root cause treatment is determinable and possible, there is an excellent opportunity for a patient to live without the fear of relapse.

Myth #6: There is no cure for bipolar disorder.

This myth comes down to the concept of cure versus propensity, and it is controversial. Most psychiatrists will tell you that you must take psychotropic medication for the rest of your life because you have the propensity, to get sick again. I think this theory is predicated on fear and flies in the face of soul contracts. My goal in working with patients is to have them take the minimum necessary dose of a nutraceutical or pharmaceutical for maximum benefit. If you can develop self-awareness, understand your triggers, manage your stress, balance your hormones, eat a healthy diet, commit to the steps outlined in this book, and, ultimately, accept yourself, I feel it is possible for you to live with little to no medication if you have bipolar disorder. Am I recommending this for you? Not necessarily. Am I suggesting that it is possible? Yes, if you do all that I have suggested in this book. I feel the propensity to experience mania, anxiety or depression is something that needs to be carefully managed. I choose to no longer live in fear of this happening it to me. Instead, I accept my experiences as part of my journey.

Myth #7: You are strong enough to will your way through mental illness without help.

This is a dangerous myth because it is a perfect example of the isolating, destructive, cycling thoughts that characterize mental illness. The moment when we most need help and should reach out and use resources is often the very time when a thought like this will keep us from doing so. Some people think that because it is an illness of thoughts, they will be able to cure themselves through sheer force of will. The issue is that the disease itself is distorting your thoughts. It is like fighting a raging house fire with a garden hose. The truth is that trying to think your way out of mental illness can perpetuate the spiral of self-blame and shame. The best way to deal with this is to open up to others (where appropriate), rely on available resources, and trust that others can help.

Myth #8: You create mental illness yourself through poor "mental hygiene" and bad psychological habits.

This is an example of victim-blaming. Mental illness is not a burden that you earn through bad habits. Mental health issues affect 20 to 25% of people in North America during the course of their lives. In part biochemical, situational, psychological, genetic, hormonal and environmental, they cannot be attributed to a single cause, and certainly not to one that we create ourselves. Developing good mental thought practices and habits, and being aware of harmful thought patterns and behaviours, is helpful. As outlined in this book, practising the Seven Rs of working with problematic thoughts and breaking the thought–emotion cycle are important steps to incorporate into your life to regain your mental health. However, these are just two of the many ways that treatment can help.

Myth #9: Mental illness is the result of a traumatic childhood and cannot be undone.

While mental illness has been associated with childhood trauma, it is absolutely not 100% causal. It is possible and very likely that you can work through and overcome the effect of childhood trauma on your adult psychological status. Holding on to the belief that something has been broken and cannot be fixed is another example of closed, negative and absolutist thinking. Statistics show that mental illness associated with trauma, abuse, neglect and many other negative experiences can be treated successfully.

Myth #10: Because mental illness is largely genetic, there is very little you can do to prevent or treat it.

Mental illness is multifactorial. While there may be a genetic component to some forms of mental illness, this predisposition can be modulated by lifestyle, along with medical and personal choices. With the help of cognitive training, proper nutritional support, regular exercise, medical monitoring, self-awareness and many other supports, mental illness can be prevented and treated. Remember the concept of epigenetics (Chapter 9), which is concerned with factors in the environment that can turn genes on or off.

Myth #11: People will look at you differently if you reach out for help.

The fear surrounding this myth is common to many health conditions. It is the fear of being seen for who we really are and is one of the biggest obstacles to our true happiness. As a culture, we make huge efforts to always put our best face forward, showing only the happy/desirable/ social-media-appropriate sides of ourselves while hiding, shaming and disowning the shadow sides. This keeps us from having true connection. Tragically, it is what keeps us from ever feeling truly loved. How can we believe that we are truly loved (all parts of us) if we never show ourselves? When we get positive feedback on the groomed face we use for the world, we reinforce the belief that the ungroomed face would not be accepted and that we must keep up our efforts to stay presentable. Mental illness thrives on this fear. The truth, however, is powerfully contradictory.

There is strength, courage and beauty in being able to show all parts of oneself, though it is uncomfortable.

Think about the last time a person truly opened up to you about something painful, and you saw that they had acknowledged it, were working toward accepting it, and were trying to love themselves and others despite their perceived "flaw." What did you feel for that person? I'm guessing it was compassion, and possibly some frustration that they should have to deal with such stress. Probably you also wished they could see themselves as you see them. Whenever I was brave enough to share my diagnosis of bipolar disorder with someone, I often expected judgment, collapse of social status, loss of friendship, misunderstanding, perhaps pity or a permanent shameful mark on my identity. When this did happen (it wasn't the norm), I have come to understand that this type of response says more about the other person's lack of compassion and understanding than it does about me.

When we see someone who is baring all, asking for help and reaching out, we are witnessing an act of vulnerability. Dr. Brené Brown is a research professor at the University of Houston Graduate College of Social Work who has spent the past 13 years studying vulnerability, courage, worthiness and shame. Vulnerability, as Dr. Brown says, is the best measure of our courage. By reaching out, you give permission to others to be more honest with the world as well. It is an example of how we can be more real with each other. Perhaps the best way to debunk this myth is by talking about it. If you are dealing with mental health concerns and you reach out for help and are seen for all you are, shadow and light, people will see you as strong enough to show, admit, accept and work with all parts of yourself. They will watch and say, "That is a whole person." And they will be emboldened to do the same for themselves.

Myth #12: You will develop a tolerance to medication and keep needing more and stronger drugs.

There is a fear that the medications used to treat psychosis, bipolar disorder, depression and anxiety are addictive. It is thought that they cause changes in the brain and body that make it very difficult to reduce or eliminate their use. Like many other medications, the body becomes accustomed to the effects of the drugs and can even begin to respond less to the drug itself, creating a type of tolerance. The thought is that once the brain adjusts to having more serotonin and less neurotransmitter breakdown, it will be unable to make enough on its own. Also, once a drug becomes less effective, patients can be switched to new or more potent medications, making it seem like once you've started, you never stop but, rather, are cycled through various forms of the same drug.

It is true that some medications can cause accommodation that may lead to withdrawal when the dosage is changed. But this doesn't mean reducing or stopping the medication is impossible. Many people do not experience any withdrawal symptoms whatsoever. For others, it is a transient biochemical adjustment that can be short-lived when supported with naturopathic medicine.

Myth #13: People with mental health issues are sick for life and will never again be reliable, functioning members of society/healthy people/good parents/teachers or other professionals.

This is an example of the kind of defeated, distorted thinking that characterizes many mental illnesses. Not only is it possible for those who deal with mental health concerns to regain full and healthy lives, but living through the experience can help them to have a better, more complete understanding of themselves and others.

Myth #14: Mental health issues affect only a small number of very unstable people.

Mental health issues will affect one in four people worldwide, according to the World Health Organization. This is a huge proportion of the global population. Mental illness can affect people from all walks of life—people who have experienced hardship or good fortune, who have healthy personal histories or who don't, who are externally "all put together" or who struggle with daily tasks. It is definitely not limited to a small number of visibly unstable people.

Myth #15: Suicide only happens when people really have no way out.

Suicide can happen when a person's mental status is so disturbed that they *believe* they have no other way out. For a suicidal person, the conclusion that there is no way out is not based on a factual observation of the world or their position and opportunities in it. Their views and decisions are coloured by "wearing dark-coloured glasses" that distort, twist and darken what is before them. There is always a way out. It is just very hard to see one when you are plagued by thoughts of suicide. Therefore, it is imperative to learn how to manage your mind so that suicide becomes a reminder of how you are being unkind and unloving to yourself in that moment, rather than a rational thought or emotion to act upon.

Myth #16: People who commit suicide are selfish.

Many people who have never experienced mental illness have a difficult time understanding why someone would want to take their own life. They view suicide as selfish because it hurts those left behind. What I think is important to understand is that suicide can be a way of relieving one's pain and suffering. I know for myself, I was so tormented by my thoughts that I determined that suicide was the only way I would be free of them. In essence, the pain I was in trumped any thoughts I had about how my death would impact others. At those low points, I felt like people would be better off if I wasn't around, as then I would no longer be a burden. I realize that this is not true, now that I practise the Seven Rs of working with problematic thoughts and breaking the thought–emotion cycle.

Myth #17: People with mental illness are dangerous or violent.

The media and movies often portray those with mental illness as violent. When exposed to these stories with no further understanding of what mental illness is, many people develop stereotypes of people with mental illness as being violent. While it is true that some individuals with mental illness can be violent, the percentage is no larger than in the general population. Researchers agree that mental illnesses are not a good predictor of violence. In fact, most of the violence surrounding mental illness throughout history has been aimed at the individual who is ill, not the other way around. Also, most people with mental illness are more dangerous to themselves than to others. I know for myself, when deciding to attempt suicide, I was extremely preoccupied with whether or not I would implicate anyone else in the process. I was so concerned about protecting my family, loved ones, innocent people and health workers that my options were extremely limited. The last thing I wanted was to inflict harm, danger or inconvenience on anyone else.

Myth #18: You are weak for not being able to overcome what you are going through. You are lazy. What you are experiencing is not real; you need to grow up.

Mental illness can be difficult to understand for those who have never been through it. Some would characterize it as an invisible disability, in that you can look at someone with mental illness and not know that they are ill. When people can't see the "disability," they have a difficult time believing it is real or that it is affecting the individual's life in any real way. Therefore, if someone is suffering from depression and is unable to "fight" or "beat" their emotional issues, others may view them as weak or lazy. What is important to understand is that laziness or lack of motivation is a symptom of depression; it is not who you are fundamentally as a person. You are not weak or lazy; you are depressed. Since mental illness affects an individual's thoughts and behaviours, it is difficult for many people to understand that this is an illness and not a choice.

Myth #19: People with depression are always sad.

If you look at almost any picture depicting someone with depression, you will see them holding their head in their hands. While it is true that feeling sad is one of the primary criteria for depression, there are many other ways in which an individual with depression is affected. The *Diagnostic and Statistical Manual* indicates that at least five of following must be present in the individual for a diagnosis to be made:

- Depressed mood most of the day, nearly every day, as indicated by either subjective report (e.g., feels sad or empty) or observation made by others (e.g., appears tearful). Note: In children and adolescents, can be irritable mood.
- Markedly diminished interest or pleasure in all, or almost all, activities most of the day, nearly every day (as indicated by either subjective account or observation made by others).
- Significant weight loss when not dieting or weight gain (e.g., a change of more than 5% of body weight in a month) or decrease or increase in appetite nearly every day. Note: In children, consider failure to make expected weight gains.
- Insomnia or hypersomnia nearly every day.
- Psychomotor agitation or retardation nearly every day (observable by others, not merely subjective feelings of restlessness or being slowed down).
- Fatigue or loss of energy nearly every day.
- Feelings of worthlessness or excessive or inappropriate guilt (which

may be delusional) nearly every day (not merely self-reproach or guilt about being sick).
- Diminished ability to think or concentrate, or indecisiveness, nearly every day (either by subjective account or as observed by others).
- Recurrent thoughts of death (not just fear of dying), recurrent suicidal ideation without a specific plan, or a suicide attempt or a specific plan for committing suicide.

Myth #20: You are your illness or the label placed on you.
This myth speaks to the title of this book. I want you to understand that you are not your label(s). In order to realize you're not, you need to look beyond many of the treatment models for mental illness, which are illness-centred as opposed to person-centred. This being the case, many practitioners do not consider who you are as a person when they offer treatment. This model reinforces that your primary identity is now your mental illness, and the care you receive will reflect this. The chart on the next page contrasts person-centred and illness-centred care in a variety of facets.

Indeed, this is the focus of this book: that you are more than the label you've been given. I no longer let bipolar disorder, bulimia, depression, anxiety or social phobia define who I am as a human being. I am no longer limited by these labels and have moved beyond them, challenging the conventional wisdom and leading a life that balances the two paradigms of medicine—Western and naturopathic.

Myth #21: Your mental health issues are completely negative; there is no gift in them.
While there is danger in romanticizing mental illness, there is also danger in ignoring the experience of it and what gifts there are in the process of recovery. Recovery is hard work and is different for everyone; but it often involves lots of self-reflection and time spent caring for oneself. This ultimately leads to a richer and more fulfilling inner life. In addition, there are countless links between mental illness and creativity; anecdotally, it seems many writers, painters, scientists and poets have had a mental illness. While it is not known whether one contributes to the other, they are seen to be related.

Here is a list of a few well-known artistically inclined people who have been diagnosed with major depressive disorder or bipolar disorder (type

PERSON-CENTRED CARE	ILLNESS-CENTRED CARE
The relationship is the foundation	The diagnosis is the foundation
Validates the person's distress	Pathologizes distress
Begin with welcoming—outreach and engagement	Begin with illness assessment
Services are based on personal suffering and help needed	Services are based on diagnosis and treatment needed
Services work toward quality-of-life goals	Services work toward illness reduction goals
Treatment and rehabilitation are goal-driven	Treatment is symptom-driven; rehabilitation is disability-driven
Personal recovery is central from beginning to end	Illness and disability are prioritized over personal recovery
Track personal progress toward recovery	Track illness progress toward symptom reduction and cure
Use techniques that promote personal growth and self-responsibility	Use techniques that promote illness control and reduction of risk
Services end when the person manages their own life and attains meaningful roles	Services end when the illness is cured

1 or 2): Russell Brand, Florence Nightingale, Winston Churchill, Carrie Fisher, Mel Gibson, Ernest Hemingway, Robert Munsch, Friedrich Nietzsche, Edgar Allan Poe, Margaret Trudeau, Ted Turner, Vincent van Gogh, Robin Williams and Virginia Woolf.

Myth #22: Antidepressants will make you fat, tired and lazy.

Weight gain and decreased energy resulting in fatigue are common side effects of some antidepressants. But not everyone who takes these medications experiences them.

Myth #23: When you are on antidepressants, you are not yourself. You are a robot, or feel "drugged up."

Some older antidepressants, such as Paxil, were known to have the side effect of causing people to feel numb. However, many newer antidepressants don't have this side effect. Many people can function at a high level while on them.

Conclusion

*"There are many roads to wellness. The important thing is to
pick a path and follow it wholeheartedly."*

DR. CHRIS

A̲T THE END of the day, all we have is love. We enter the world with
nothing but love and excitement for our arrival. The key is to
take all the love that has ever been felt for us and direct that not
only inward to ourselves, but outward—to bring joy and love to every situation we encounter. When I have been depressed, it has been like my
love light gets turned off and the replacement battery is lost. But that is
the journey we are on—to return to the place of love for ourselves, for
each other and for the planet.

The word "normal" doesn't always help us ignite the love we have
for ourselves, especially when we feel or are told that we aren't normal
and have a mental illness. What I find with any mental health state outside the realm of what society deems "normal" is that everyone (family
members, doctors, therapists, nurses) is trying to get the person *out* of
that state versus teaching them to *accept*, *understand* and *love* all aspects
of themselves, including that state. In my opinion, we need to expand
our definition of normal and perhaps embrace the lessons that might be
found in the fringes of our mind.

Phrases like "This moment has gone wrong," "This is not the path,"
"There is something wrong with me," or "This should not be happening"
are at the core of suffering. We need to look at our suffering as an invitation to meet ourselves in a way that we've never met ourselves before.
The sense around our suffering is that we can't do this, but we forget our

vast nature and the concept of soul contracts. The experience we are having is here because we are here. It is important to look at it all as sacred and part of our journey to wellness. All your thoughts, feelings and sensations appear in your presence. It is your presence that is the constant in your life. Feelings can surge up and thoughts can explode like fireworks, but they all fall back into you. You are the root and the birthplace of your thoughts, feelings and sensations. With each breath of awareness, we can rest in acceptance of the vastness of who we are.

Remember that even the darkest parts of ourselves—the parts that we don't like, love or accept—are a call for love. These aspects of ourselves only seem dark because we haven't shone the light of love on them. Every day, we are invited by life to turn to this moment and accept it just as it is. Something is trying to break out, break free or be born in someone who is struggling. In our suffering, we often feel alone. With mental illness, we always seem to be running away from it, trying to fix it, trying to get rid of it, and in these efforts, we end up ignoring the present moment. Remember that life is here. It is in the breath, in this feeling of sadness, this feeling of joy—it is all inclusive. This moment, whatever shape it takes, is all there is now. To be open to life, we need to see it as sacred. That means letting go of our expectations about how we thought this moment was supposed to look.

No one knows how long they have on Earth—life is fragile, precious, a gift and can be gone in the blink of an eye. Pema Chodron wrote:

Sometimes impermanence smacks us in the face without much warning. It was always there, of course, lurking in the background, we've just been distracted, or fallen into illusions of permanence.... And then, a cancer diagnosis. Loss of livelihood, wealth, power. The unexpected end of a relationship. A broken promise, a shattered dream. These are not mistakes or punishments but sudden reminders of the sheer Power of the Uncontrollable, the immense Intelligence moving all things, an Intelligence beyond comprehension ... an invitation to remember: in the midst of cancer, loss, devastation, failure, what cannot be lost? What cannot fail? Love is still here. The ability to connect deeply. To listen. To see. To feel. To laugh at seriousness. To be serious about laughter. To remember our own Presence, the Presence of life, here and now. And the gift of the small things. The breath moving through the nostrils. A visit from a loved one. An unspoken kindness. The beauty of questions unanswered.... This is not a path you will find in books. This is a path of courage and birdsong, of waking in the morning with a tender heart and knowing that everything is somehow profoundly okay in a way you cannot hope to understand.

I know it is not easy to understand mental illness, and you can get trapped in asking "Why? Why? *Why*? Why *me*?" But all we have is this moment. This breath. Now. My hope is that you will use the steps outlined in this book—starting where you feel is right for you and continuing through each step as needed.

Since I struggled with my mental health in my childhood, as an adolescent and into adulthood, my passion in life has become to authentically share my experiences and what I have been through to help others regain their mental health. On the one hand, I have been treated like a criminal—disrespectfully and abusively by police—mistaken for a homeless person, judged, afraid to say anything about my diagnosis, shut out by family members, and unforgiven for things I've done or said while in the depths of psychosis or completely mad. I've lost friendships; I've escaped from the hospital and almost been reported as a missing person; I've had my father lock me out of his house and call the police because my stepmother was afraid of me. I've been locked in a police holding cell when I refused hospital admission.

And on the other hand, I've been so loved by my parents, granny, husband, aunt and uncle, many cousins and friends—all of whom understood the masks of mental illness. They have allowed my beauty to prevail through my darkest struggles. They have not given up. They have not abandoned me in my hours of need. For those who have, all I can do is ask forgiveness, pray for compassion and hope they will learn to give mental health the love and understanding it deserves. Remember, the person is still there, even in the throes of psychosis or the depths of depression. There is a human being in there. Be kind. Be compassionate. Reach them.

My ascents into madness and descents back into depression have been extremely painful experiences. They have also been completely misunderstood by society and, unfortunately, by police. And I'm not alone: my patients have been tasered by police because they were psychotic and defying orders. Many police officers think we are on drugs. I hope this book serves as an agent of change to create more understanding, awareness and compassion in that profession as well as in society in general.

Now that I am "almost" on the other side of my struggles, I wouldn't change any experience I have had, no matter how painful it has been, because it has shaped me into the person I am today. I want you to know that your journey is sacred, even if you feel there is no hope. My prayer is that you will benefit from reading about my experiences and turn toward life to accept this moment—whatever shape it takes.

I used quotations above around the word "almost" because I truly feel that we are all works in progress. Although I am respected for my work in the naturopathic mental health field, my ego knows that labels like "expert," "the best," and so on are just that—labels.

As a recovering "type A perfectionist," I recently read Brené Brown's book *The Gifts of Imperfection*, and it got me thinking about the difference between wanting to be perfect and wanting to be the best. I feel there is a difference. Initially, in my teenage and early adulthood years, I think I was more focused on being perfect, never letting anyone see me make a mistake because on a fundamental level I was trying to measure up and earn my place in society. But there is a grey area where the drive to be the best crosses into the danger zone of perfection or addiction. For me, this internal drive to be the best stems from being adopted, since I never felt worthy, loved or wanted and always set the bar high for myself.

As I have regained my mental health, overcome my body and eating issues, and come to understand myself, I see that this has shifted for me. Now the driving force in my life is about being the best I can be as a human being versus being perfect. Now I take a much more balanced approach to life and health by always considering the mental, emotional and spiritual aspects of my life. I think this is a subtle but important distinction.

⟶ *In your **Moving Beyond** journal, answer the following questions:*

· *In what areas of your life do you strive to improve?*
· *Reflect on the difference between being perfect and being the best. Which word resonates more with you, and why?*
· *Is there an area in your life that is bordering on unhealthy for you in terms of striving to be perfect or the best?*

WHAT DO I WANT?

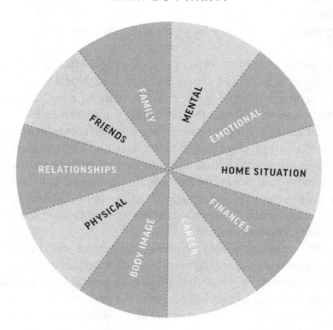

A useful tool to bring more balance into your life and guide you in the direction of change is to complete the "What do I want?" exercise above. Spend some time thinking about what you want in 10 key areas of your life. As you fill in the circle above, think of it as a wheel that has to roll down a hill. If you are a 10/10 in your career, but a 2/10 in your body image, then the wheel is uneven, and it won't roll very well. Consider the gaps in your life and contemplate how you can address them to bring lasting joy and happiness into your life.

🔑 *In your **Moving Beyond** journal, complete the "What do I want?" exercise by asking yourself what your desires are in the areas listed.*

Since starting my journey in naturopathic medicine, I have had:

- *Much better quality of life, to the point where I now enjoy life versus continually wanting to end it, as I did in the past*
- *An improvement in my health to the point of rarely needing mood stabilizing medications, given my ability to blend naturopathic and Western medicine. (It is important to reiterate that I am not anti-medication, but*

I am in favour of minimum dose for maximum benefit. I also feel that addressing the mental, emotional and spiritual aspects of health is at least as important as addressing the physical aspect, if not more so.)

As a health care practitioner, I do not judge, label, pigeon-hole or classify people as the medical profession likes to. Nor do I say to people, "one complaint per visit." I believe that to truly be a helpful servant to my patients, I need to listen to them; fully understand the life circumstances that brought them to where they are; address their shadow and core beliefs through cognitive behavioural and compassion-focused therapy; help them make dietary changes so they have the nutritional building blocks to support the formation of hormones and neurotransmitters; address the stressful situations in their lives that may be keeping them stuck; and teach them mindfulness tools to handle stress so they can live their lives to the fullest.

The most important voice you have is that of your intuition. By practising the Seven Rs of working with problematic thoughts and breaking the thought–emotion cycle, you will learn to trust your inner voice over that of your ego. Remember that "What we resist persists," so it is critical to become an objective observer of your subjective mind. Become curious about your thoughts instead of suppressing them. Acknowledge them and thank them for coming to teach you a lesson, ask them what they have come to teach you and then *stop*, connect with your breath and send the healing energy of the breath to areas in your body that need healing. Pause long enough to allow yourself to hear the answers from your body. It is only when we are calm and quiet in our minds that we can hear our inner voices and realize the personal truths that reside inside us. It takes time. It takes practice. It takes patience. These are all available to you right away. Get started now. Take one small step in support of you, today. Make your life matter. Don't be afraid to let your light shine. I know that you are here for a reason.

Naturopathic medicine is about health promotion and prevention as well as correcting imbalances in the body. For me, taking a balanced approach to health is the best form of medicine. Remember that health is a journey, not a destination. Ultimately, we all want to be at the destination of optimal health yesterday. The reality is that the road to recovery may be full of potholes—or perhaps trees need to chopped down and the ground levelled before the road can be paved. Regardless, it is important that you take the first step. Doing nothing is not the best option if you are suffering. If you have been recently diagnosed, or are struggling in any way, please accept my helping hand offered in the steps outlined in this book. Let them guide you to optimum health. Have faith that you can get well. I believe you can, and I wish you all the joy there is to be found on the healing journey. Let love for yourself and others always be your guide.

Eating for Mental Wellness

THIS APPENDIX contains three subsections aimed at helping you eat in a way that supports your mental wellness. The sections are:

1. **Top 10 Food Sources of the Essential Nutrients**—Lists of the top 10 foods containing nutrients, from vitamin A to zinc and many others.

2. **The Dirty Dozen Endocrine Disruptors**—A chart listing the worst hormone disruptors, what they do, and how to avoid them.

3. **Mental Health Diet**—A handy chart suggesting meals and snacks each day for two weeks, followed by the recipes you need to follow the plan.

Best Sources of Essential Nutrients

TOP 10 FOODS CONTAINING OMEGA 3 ESSENTIAL FATTY ACIDS

Food	Amount	mg
Flaxseed oil	5 ml	2,580
Chia seeds (dried)	15 ml	1,900
Wild Atlantic salmon	100 g	2,586

Mackerel (cooked)	100 g	2,070
Trout	100 g	1,370
Nutrasea fish oil	5 ml	1,250
Cod liver oil	5 ml	888
Mackerel (salted)	100 g	5,134
Sockeye salmon	100 g	2,865
Walnuts (chopped)	28 g	2,565

TOP 10 FOODS RICH IN VITAMIN B6

Food	Amount	mg
Bluefin tuna (cooked)	100 g	0.5
Wheat bran	28 g	0.4
Ground turkey (cooked)	1 patty (81 g)	0.3
Spinach (cooked)	100 g	0.2
Prunes	28 g	0.2
Beef liver (pan fried)	1 slice (81 g)	0.8
Banana	1 medium	0.4
Pistachios (roasted, unsalted)	28 g	0.4
Avocado	½ medium	0.3
Sunflower seeds, dry roasted	1 oz.	0.2

TOP 10 FOOD SOURCES OF TRYPTOPHAN

Food	Amount	mg
Cottage cheese, 2% fat	250 ml	400
Beef liver	85 g	334
Peanuts	85 g	291
Lamb, leg roast	85 g	283
Turkey	85 g	283
Canned tuna	85 g	270
Beef, chuck	85 g	260
Salmon	85 g	231
Wild game	85 g	230
Cashews	20 whole	215

TOP 10 FOOD SOURCES OF VITAMIN C

Food	Amount	mg
Peppers (red, yellow) (raw)	125 ml	144
Peppers (red, green) (cooked)	125 ml	132
Green peppers	125 ml	96
Pepper, red chili	1 pepper	109
Broccoli (cooked)	125 ml	54
Cabbage (red) (raw)	250 ml	54
Brussel sprouts (cooked)	4 sprouts	73
Kohlrabi (cooked)	125 ml	47
Broccoli (raw)	125 ml	66
Snow peas (cooked)	125 ml	41

TOP 10 FOOD SOURCES OF MAGNESIUM

Food	Amount	mg
Soybean flour	125 ml	310
Buckwheat flour	125 ml	246
Cereal, Raisin Bran	30 g	144
Soybeans, dried	250 ml	138
Whole-wheat flour	125 ml	136
Tofu, firm	250 ml	118
Cheerios	250 ml	117
Rye	100 g	102
Figs (dried)	250 ml	100
Black-eyed peas (cooked)	250 ml	98

TOP 10 FOOD SOURCES OF ZINC

Food	Amount	mg
Oysters (Eastern)	75 g	59
Oysters (Pacific)	75 g	33
Liver, veal (cooked)	75 g	8.5
Beef, roast	75 g	5.3
Baked beans, cooked	175 ml	4.3
Turkey, dark meat	75 g	2.7
Wheat germ (toasted)	30 ml	2.4
Cheddar cheese	100 g	3.3
Swiss cheese	100 g	3.3
Swiss chard	250 ml	3.2

TOP 10 FOOD SOURCES OF VITAMIN B12

Food	Amount	mcg
Clams (cooked)	28 g	27.7
Liver of lamb, beef and other animals	28 g	Up to 24
Mackerel (Atlantic, cooked)	100 g	19
Kellogg's All-Bran Buds (fortified)	30 g	6
Silk soymilk (fortified)	250 ml	3
Ground beef	85 g	2.4
Swiss cheese	28 g	0.9
Yogourt, plain, whole milk	113 g	0.4
Roasted chicken breast	100 g	0.3
Hard-boiled egg	1 egg	0.6

SOURCES:
Medical Nutrition from Marz by Russell Marz, ND
Textbook of Natural Medicine by Joseph Pizzorno & Michael Murray. Nutrient data was obtained from the USDA SR-21 Food composition database: ndb.nal.usda.gov/ndb/.

The Dirty Dozen Endocrine Disruptors

Here are 12 of the worst hormone disruptors, what they do, and how to avoid them.

CHEMICAL	WHAT IT DOES	WHERE IT IS FOUND
Atrazine	Feminizes male frogs.	A herbicide used on corn and other non-organic crops.
BPA (bisphenol A)	Mimics sex hormones in human body. Linked with breast and reproductive cancers. Linked with obesity, early puberty and heart disease.	In the linings of food cans, in receipt paper, and in plastics (especially plastic water bottles, anything marked PC [polycarbonate] or plastic #7).
Dioxin	Disrupts delicate signalling systems of male and female hormones. Affects immune and reproductive systems; even in utero exposure can reduce adult sperm count in men.	Animal products including meat, fish, milk, eggs and butter are most likely to be contaminated.
Perchlorate	Competes with iodine in the body, affecting thyroid hormone function.	In tap water and many food sources. Reduce its impact by making sure your salt is iodized.

CHEMICAL	WHAT IT DOES	WHERE IT IS FOUND
Phthalates	Increase death of some cells in body. Linked with low sperm count, lowered sperm motility, birth defects, obesity, diabetes, and thyroid irregularities.	In plastic food containers, children's toys, plastic wrap, makeup and other personal care products. Anything with the ingredient "fragrance" that does not say phthalate-free. Find phthalate-free personal care products with EWG's Skin Deep Database: **ewg.org/skindeep**.
Fire retardants (PDBES)	Mimic thyroid hormone and disrupt thyroid activity.	On many manufactured products: furniture, carpeting, house materials and surfaces. Reduce exposure with HEPA air filter in the home and avoid exposure to dust/chemicals during renovation.
Arsenic	Linked with skin, bladder and lung cancer. Interferes with glucocorticoid system (body's system of processing sugars and carbohydrates), leading to weight change, insulin resistance, diabetes, osteoporosis, growth retardation, high blood pressure and weakened immune system. Lethal in high amounts.	Factory farm chicken and unfiltered tap water. Use a water filter to reduce exposure. For help finding a good water filter, check out EWG's buying guide: **ewg.org/report/ewgs-water-filter-buying-guide**.

CHEMICAL	WHAT IT DOES	WHERE IT IS FOUND
Lead	Lowers sex hormones in animals (including humans). Negatively affects the body's major stress-coping system. Toxic especially to children. Can cause permanent brain damage, reduced IQ, hearing loss, miscarriage, premature birth, increased blood pressure, kidney damage, and nervous system problems, like anxiety and depression.	In old paints (prior to 1978), drinking water, old varnishes and surface finishes.
Mercury	Concentrates in the fetal brain and negatively affects brain development. Binds to sex hormones and interferes with hormone signalling. May play a role in the development of diabetes.	In seafood (particularly canned tuna), old mercury amalgam dental fillings, and some vaccinations.
Glycol ethers	May impact fertility or harm a fetus in utero. Linked with lower sperm counts and shrunken testicles in rats. May be linked with higher incidence of asthma and allergies.	In paints, cleaning products, brake fluid and cosmetics. Specifically contained in products with the ingredients 2-butoxyethanol (EGBEO) and methoxydiglycol (DEGME).

CHEMICAL	WHAT IT DOES	WHERE IT IS FOUND
Organo-phosphate pesticides	Linked with negative effects on brain development, behaviour and fertility. Lowers testosterone and affects thyroid function.	Any non-organic produce or other foods. Especially high in the EWG's Dirty Dozen list.
Perfluorinated chemicals (PFCS)	Linked with decreased sperm quality, low birth weight, kidney disease, thyroid disease, and high cholesterol. Known to affect thyroid and sex hormones in animals.	In non-stick pans and water-resistant coating on clothing, furniture and carpets.

EWG = Environmental Working Group

SOURCES:
www.ewg.org/research/dirty-dozen-list-endocrine-disruptors
www.globalresearch.ca
www.naturalnews.com/029720_hormones_health.html

Mental Health Diet

Here is a handy two-week diet plan that includes recipes for nutritional support of balanced mental health. (For a list of the recipe references, see page 359.)

WEEK 1

....

MONDAY

Breakfast	– Steel-cut oatmeal
	– Non-dairy milk
	– Organic pear
Morning Snack	– Green goddess smoothie
Lunch	– Curried chicken salad
	– Whole-grain crackers
Afternoon Snack	– ¼ cup unsalted nuts
Dinner	– Grilled salmon with balsamic onion glaze
	– Steamed kale

....

TUESDAY

Breakfast	– Warm quinoa porridge
Morning Snack	– Apple slices
	– ¼ cup pumpkin seeds
Lunch	– Lentil vegetable soup
	– Cornmeal carrot muffin
Afternoon Snack	– ¼ cup almonds
Dinner	– Ginger chicken stir fry

WEDNESDAY

Breakfast	– Blueberry buckwheat pancakes
Morning Snack	– Veggies with hummus
Lunch	– Pita sandwich
Afternoon Snack	– Organic fruit (½ to 1 cup)
Dinner	– Turkey tacos

THURSDAY

Breakfast	– ½ cantaloupe – Spelt toast with banana nut butter spread
Morning Snack	– ¼ cup unsalted mixed nuts
Lunch	– Soba noodle veggie pot
Afternoon Snack	– Krispy kale chips
Dinner	– Three-bean vegetarian chili

FRIDAY

Breakfast	– Apple and hazelnut muesli
Morning Snack	– ¼ cup unsalted mixed nuts
Lunch	– Raw pad Thai
Afternoon Snack	– Veggies with hummus
Dinner	– Vegetable lasagna

SATURDAY

Breakfast	– Blueberry hemp smoothie – Crispy breakfast bars
Morning Snack	– Organic celery sticks with almond butter
Lunch	– Cranberry quinoa salad
Afternoon Snack	– Organic fruit (½ to 1 cup)
Dinner	– Shrimp in Thai green curry with wild rice

SUNDAY

Breakfast	– ½ honeydew melon
	– Poached or hard/soft-boiled eggs
	– sausages
Morning Snack	– Organic celery sticks with almond butter
Lunch	– Garden bean soup
Afternoon Snack	– Organic zucchini sticks with lentil dip
Dinner	– Almond chicken
	– Asian asparagus

WEEK 2

MONDAY

Breakfast	– Grain-free berry muffins
	– Fresh fruit
Morning Snack	– ¼ cup trail mix
Lunch	– Ginger butternut soup
Afternoon Snack	– Veggies with hummus
Dinner	– Flax baked chicken
	– Roasted beets and spinach salad

TUESDAY

Breakfast	– Warm quinoa porridge
Morning Snack	– Organic fruit (½ to 1 cup)
Lunch	– Wonderful whatever salad (leftover chicken)
Afternoon Snack	– ¼ cup almonds
Dinner	– Vegetarian chili with avocado salsa

WEDNESDAY

Breakfast	– Berry-almond slam smoothie
Morning Snack	– ¼ cup unsalted nuts
Lunch	– Warm spicy sweet potato salad
Afternoon Snack	– Krispy kale chips
Dinner	– Sesame-seed-crusted salmon burgers with sliced avocado – Chickpea slaw

THURSDAY

Breakfast	– Blueberry buckwheat pancakes
Morning Snack	– Organic celery sticks with almond butter
Lunch	– Edamame and bean salad with shrimp and fresh salsa
Afternoon Snack	– Apple slices – Handful of pumpkin seeds
Dinner	– Spaghetti squash and black bean tacos

FRIDAY

Breakfast	– Instant flax seed cereal
Morning Snack	– ¼ cup trail mix
Lunch	– Fresh salad rolls with tangy almond dipping sauce
Afternoon Snack	– Organic zucchini sticks with lentil dip
Dinner	– Almond chicken – Stewed kale and lentils

SATURDAY

Breakfast	– Warm oat and apple bowl
Morning Snack	– Organic fruit (½ to 1 cup)
Lunch	– Arugula rainbow salad
Afternoon Snack	– ¼ cup trail mix
Dinner	– Ultimate turkey and spinach lasagna

SUNDAY

Breakfast	– Rice bread with sliced avocado
Morning Snack	– Organic celery sticks with almond butter
Lunch	– Garden bean soup
Afternoon Snack	– Organic fruit (½ to 1 cup)
Dinner	– Pumpkin-seed-crusted halibut
	– Kale salad

WEEK 1 MONDAY

Steel-Cut Oatmeal (SERVES 2)

3 C water
1 C dry organic steel-cut oats
non-dairy milk
organic pear
cinnamon

DIRECTIONS: Bring 3 cups water to a boil, add oats and reduce and cook for 20-30 minutes. Add cinnamon as oats finish cooking. Stir in non-dairy milk to taste and slice organic pear on top.

Green Goddess Smoothie (SERVES 1)

1 C frozen organic strawberries

1 orange

½ C diced fresh pineapple

1 to 3 kale leaves

1 handful spinach leaves

1 to 2 C water, rice milk or other milk substitute

1 serving protein powder that is as natural as possible, without too many additives or intense flavours (ask your ND for recommendations)

1 tbsp ground flaxseed or flaxseed oil

DIRECTIONS: Put all ingredients in a food processor, Magic Bullet or blender and pulse until smooth, adding more liquid if necessary.

Curried Chicken Salad (SERVES 4+)

2½ to 3 C (1 to 1.5 lb) chicken or turkey, cooked, cooled, and diced

1 C diced organic celery

½ C organic raisins

½ C raw almond slices

1 to 2 tsp curry powder

¼ to ½ tsp cayenne powder to taste

1 to 2 tsp apple cider vinegar

½ to 1 C mayonnaise or substitute (e.g., Community Spectrum Naturals, Veganaise). See below for Believable Vegan Mayonnaise recipe.

DIRECTIONS: Combine the chicken, celery, raisins, and almond slices in a large bowl and mix together with a large spoon. Add curry and cayenne powder and mix the ingredients together again. Drizzle on the vinegar and add the mayonnaise, starting with about ½ cup and adding more to your preference. Refrigerate for 1-2 hours before serving, to enable flavours to integrate.

Believable Vegan Mayonnaise (MAKES APPROXIMATELY ½ CUP)

4 oz silken organic tofu

2 tsp fresh organic lemon juice

1 tsp Dijon mustard

½ C oil (extra virgin olive, camelina, hemp, flax, avocado oil)

sea salt

DIRECTIONS: Combine tofu, lemon juice and mustard in a blender or with a wand blender for about 30 seconds or until the tofu is smooth. While blending, slowly add in the oil and salt until emulsified and the mixture thickens to a mayonnaise-like consistency.

Grilled Salmon with Balsamic Onion Glaze (SERVES 2)

BALSAMIC ONION GLAZE
2 tbsp olive oil
2 large onions, sliced
⅓ C balsamic vinegar
salt and pepper

SALMON
½ C balsamic vinegar
2 sprigs fresh rosemary
6 × 4-oz salmon fillet portions, pin bones removed
olive oil
salt and pepper

DIRECTIONS: For balsamic onion glaze, heat oil in a large sauté pan over medium heat and add onions. Sweat onions, stirring often, until all liquid has evaporated, about 20 minutes. Add half of balsamic vinegar and simmer until absorbed. Add remaining balsamic and reduce until a glaze. Season to taste and set aside.

For salmon, preheat a grill to medium-high. Reduce balsamic with rosemary in a small saucepot to a glaze consistency, about 8 minutes, and set aside. Brush salmon fillets lightly with olive oil and season. Grill skin-side up, for 4 minutes, then rotate 90 degrees and cook 4 more minutes. Turn salmon over and cook for 8 more minutes for medium doneness. Brush salmon with rosemary balsamic mixture during last 5 minutes of cooking. Serve salmon with balsamic onion glaze on the side.

Steamed Kale (SERVES 4)

1 bunch kale, stems removed, chopped
juice of 1 lemon
2 to 3 tbsp olive oil
sea salt

DIRECTIONS: Steam kale until tender, approximately 3 minutes. Dress with lemon juice, olive oil and sea salt. Swiss chard and mustard greens can be prepared and dressed the same way.

WEEK 1 TUESDAY

Warm Quinoa Porridge (SERVES 2)

2 C filtered water
¾ C rolled quinoa flakes
1 tsp cinnamon
½ tsp cardamom powder
¼ tsp nutmeg
¼ tsp turmeric
1 tbsp raw honey OR 5 drops stevia extract liquid
sea salt
½ C diced apple
½ C blueberries (if frozen, add before quinoa to thaw)
¼ C chopped almonds or hemp seeds

DIRECTIONS: Boil water in a small saucepan. Add the rolled quinoa and stir for 2 to 3 minutes. Remove from heat and mix in the spices, raw honey, apple, blueberries and almonds.

Lentil Vegetable Soup (SERVES 6)
*Prepare night before (2-hr prep)

2 C lentils
8 C filtered water
2 C organic chicken broth
½ C chopped onion
½ C chopped organic celery
¼ C chopped organic carrot
3 tbsp organic parsley
1 clove garlic
2 tsp salt

¼ tsp pepper

½ tsp organic oregano

1 tbsp Worcestershire sauce

1 x 28-oz can diced tomatoes

2 tbsp apple cider vinegar

DIRECTIONS: Rinse lentils and place in a large soup pot. Add water and chicken broth and the remaining ingredients except tomatoes and vinegar. Cover and simmer for 1½ hours. Add tomatoes and vinegar and simmer for ½ hour more.

Cornmeal Carrot Muffins (MAKES 12)

1 C flour blend—rice, quinoa, buckwheat etc.

¾ C coarsely ground cornmeal

1 tsp baking soda

1 tsp baking powder

½ tsp salt

½ C brown sugar

2 large eggs

½ C organic canola oil

½ C rice milk

1½ C grated carrots

DIRECTIONS: Preheat oven to 350 F. Line a 12-cup muffin tin with paper liners. Combine the flour blend, cornmeal, baking soda, baking powder, and salt in a medium bowl and set aside. Whisk the eggs and the brown sugar in a large bowl until frothy. Add the oil and milk and whisk to combine. Stir in the carrots and then the dry mixture, and mix until no flour clumps remain. Divide the batter evenly between the muffin cups and bake 20 to 25 minutes. Cool 5 minutes, then transfer muffins to wire rack to cool completely before serving.

Ginger Chicken Stir Fry (SERVES 2)

4 baby bok choy

3 skinless, boneless organic free-range chicken breasts

½ C teriyaki sauce

3 tbsp cornstarch

1 tsp grated fresh ginger

1 clove garlic

1 tbsp coconut oil

1 C organic, low-sodium chicken broth

4 C spinach, lightly packed

DIRECTIONS: Slice baby bok choy in half lengthwise. Cut chicken into bite-size strips. In a bowl, stir teriyaki and cornstarch until dissolved. Add garlic and ginger. Heat oil in a large frying pan or wok over medium-high heat. Add chicken and stir fry until no longer pink, about 3 minutes. Add broth, teriyaki mixture and bok choy. Stir constantly until chicken is cooked through, 3-4 minutes. Stir in spinach and serve over brown or wild rice.

WEEK 1 WEDNESDAY
....

Blueberry Buckwheat Pancakes (SERVES 2)

¾ C light or dark buckwheat flour

½ tsp cinnamon

¼ tsp sea salt

1 C fresh or frozen blueberries

3 tbsp unsweetened rice or almond milk

3 tbsp water

2 tbsp sunflower oil

½ tsp vanilla extract

1 flax egg replacer*

*To make the egg replacer, combine 1 tablespoon of ground flaxseed with 3 tablespoons of water and let sit for 2 minutes.

DIRECTIONS: Stir the flour, cinnamon and salt together in a medium mixing bowl. Stir in the blueberries. Combine the milk, water, 1 tablespoon of the sunflower oil, and the vanilla in a small bowl. Stir the flax egg replacer into the milk mixture. Pour the milk mixture into the flour mixture, mixing until just combined, using a whisk if necessary. If the batter is too stiff, add a little more milk. Heat the remaining 1 tablespoon of sunflower oil on a griddle or in a frying pan over medium-low heat, and then pour 2 tablespoons of the batter onto the griddle, making 4 pancakes. Buckwheat flour browns quickly, so make sure the griddle or pan is not too hot. Once the edges are slightly browned and a few bubbles have formed on top, flip the pancakes over to cook the other side.

Hummus (MAKES 4 SERVINGS, OR APPROXIMATELY 1 CUP)
*Make enough to use in your pita sandwich at lunch.

1 15-oz can chickpeas, drained and rinsed
2 cloves garlic, coarsely chopped
1 tbsp tahini (sesame seed butter)
juice of 1 small lemon
1 tsp dried parsley
1 tsp paprika
½ tsp sea salt
1 tsp freshly ground pepper
¼ C extra virgin olive oil

DIRECTIONS: In a food processor, combine the chickpeas, garlic, tahini, lemon juice, parsley, paprika, salt and pepper. Pulse until combined.

With the processor running, slowly add the olive oil through the feed tube, continually pulsing until mixture is smooth. If the hummus is still chunky, add some of the reserved chickpea liquid and process until hummus is smooth.

Pita Sandwich (SERVES 1)

1 medium rice pita
turkey, sliced
hummus (recipe above)
½ C sprouts
4 slices tomato
2–3 lettuce leaves

DIRECTIONS: Slice one end of the pita so it creates a pouch. Spread hummus throughout the pita and fill pita with toppings.

Turkey Tacos (SERVES 4)

Jack's taco seasoning (recipe below)
1 tsp olive oil
1 lb ground lean turkey
¾ C water
whole-wheat tortillas, sour cream, guacamole, diced scallions, and tomatoes
    (optional)

DIRECTIONS: Heat the olive oil in a large skillet over medium-high heat. Break up the ground turkey into small pieces and cook thoroughly (5 minutes). Drain the fat and reduce the heat. Add the taco seasoning mix (recipe below) and water, then stir to blend the spices with the meat. Reduce the heat to a simmer. Serve on tortilla, with diced scallions, tomatoes, sour cream and guacamole.

Jack's Taco Seasoning (SERVES 4)

1 tsp ground cumin
1 tsp ground oregano
½ tsp onion powder
½ tsp garlic powder
½ tsp paprika
¼ to ½ tsp ground cayenne pepper
¼ to ½ tsp cayenne pepper flakes

DIRECTIONS: Mix ingredients together, adding cayenne to taste.

WEEK 1 THURSDAY

Banana Nut Butter Spread (MAKES ¾ TO 1 CUP)

1 medium banana (can be frozen)
2 to 4 tbsp organic peanut butter, depending on taste
    (or almond, cashew, pumpkin seed butter, etc.)
½ tsp cinnamon
¼ tsp organic vanilla (optional)

DIRECTIONS: Whisk ingredients in a food processor or blender until smooth. Leftovers can be stored in the fridge. Enjoy on spelt toast with half cantaloupe.

Soba Noodle Veggie Pot (SERVES 4)

1 head green or purple cabbage
1 tbsp organic extra virgin olive oil
1 C thinly sliced onion
1 C julienned carrot
1 tsp sea salt or pink rock salt, divided
½ package 100% buckwheat soba noodles
2 cloves garlic, minced

DRESSING
1 tbsp raw honey
2 tbsp miso
1 tbsp toasted sesame oil
½ C pumpkin seeds
½ tsp umeboshi plum paste (optional)

DIRECTIONS: Slice cabbage into thin strips to make 3 cups, set aside. Heat olive oil in a large skillet over medium-low heat, sauté onion until tender, about 5 minutes. Add cabbage, carrots and salt, stirring until cabbage is well coated. Reduce heat to medium-low. Cover and cook for 20 minutes, stirring occasionally, until cabbage is very tender. Meanwhile, bring 4 L of filtered water to a boil in a large pot. Add the noodles and ½ tsp salt. Boil until al dente, about 6 minutes. Whisk dressing ingredients together and set aside. Drain noodles and rinse under warm running water. Toss noodles with the vegetable mixture and dressing. Serve and top with pumpkin seeds.

Krispy Kale Chips (2–4 SERVINGS)

2 bunches green curly kale, washed, large stem removed, torn into bite-sized pieces

"CHEESE" COATING
1 C unsalted cashews, soaked 2 hrs
1 C grated sweet potato
1 lemon, juiced (about 4 tbsp)

2 tbsp nutritional yeast

1 tbsp raw honey

½ tsp sea salt or pink rock salt

2 tbsp filtered water

DIRECTIONS: Place kale in large mixing bowl. Blend remaining ingredients in a blender until smooth. Pour over kale and mix thoroughly with your hands to coat (you want it to be really glued on to the kale.) Place kale onto unbleached parchment paper and dehydrate for 6 hours at 115 F. You'll need to use 2 trays. If you don't own a dehydrator, set your oven to 150 F and dehydrate for 2 hours. Turn leaves after 1 hour to ensure even drying. Remove and store in a dry, airtight container.

Three-Bean Vegetarian Chili (SERVES 4)

3 tbsp extra virgin olive oil

1 C chopped onion

2 tsp ground cumin

1 tsp crushed red pepper

1 tsp paprika

¼ tsp salt

4 cloves garlic, thinly sliced

2 C organic vegetable broth

1½ C of ½-inch cubed peeled butternut squash

1 28-oz can diced tomatoes

1 15-oz can pinto beans, rinsed and drained

1 15-oz can cannellini beans, rinsed and drained

1 15-oz can red kidney beans, rinsed and drained

½ C thinly sliced green onion

DIRECTIONS: Add oil to pan; swirl to coat. Add onion; cook 5 minutes, stirring occasionally. Stir in cumin, red pepper, paprika, salt and garlic cloves; cook 2 minutes; stirring frequently. Add broth, squash, and tomatoes; bring to a simmer. Cook 20 minutes, stirring occasionally. Add beans; simmer 25 minutes or until slightly thick, stirring occasionally. Sprinkle with green onions.

WEEK 1 FRIDAY

....

Apple and Hazelnut Muesli (SERVES 4)

½ C rolled oats

½ C dried apricots, chopped

½ C toasted hazelnuts, chopped roughly

½ C fresh apple juice

½ C filtered water

2 apples, peeled and grated

1 tbsp maple syrup (optional)

DIRECTIONS: In a large bowl, mix together oats, apricots and hazelnuts. Pour over the apple juice and leave for 10 minutes to allow the oats and dried fruit to soak up the juice. Divide the muesli between 4 bowls and top with grated apple. Optional to drizzle maple syrup on top. Serve immediately.

Raw Pad Thai (SERVES 2-4)

1 medium zucchini

1 large carrot

1 green onion, chopped

½ C shredded purple cabbage

½ C cauliflower florets

½ C mung beans sprouts or radish sprouts (spicy)

SAUCE

2 tbsp tahini

2 tbsp almond butter

1 tbsp lime or lemon juice

2 tbsp tamari (wheat-free)

1 tbsp raw honey

¼ tsp minced garlic

½ tsp grated ginger root

DIRECTIONS: Use a spiralizer or mandolin or vegetable peeler to create noodles from carrots and zucchini. Place them in a large mixing bowl and top with the vegetables. Whisk sauce ingredients in a bowl. The sauce will be thick, but will thin out after its mixed with the vegetables. Pour the sauce over the noodles and vegetables and toss. This dish tastes even better the next day, once the flavours have had a chance to blend.

Hummus

See Week 1 Wednesday for recipe.

Vegetable Lasagna (SERVES 8)

1½ C raw cashews

sea salt

12 brown rice lasagna noodles

2 × ¼ C olive oil, divided

1 white or yellow onion, diced

1 small eggplant, peeled and diced

1 lb mushrooms, cleaned and sliced

1 red bell pepper, seeded and chopped

4 cloves garlic, minced, divided

28-oz can diced tomatoes

½ tsp black pepper

¼ tsp crushed red pepper flakes

2 tsp dried basil

2 tsp dried oregano

1 tsp fresh lemon juice

2 tsp nutritional yeast

1 C fresh basil leaves

DIRECTIONS: Soak cashews in filtered water for 2–24 hours. Drain and set aside. Boil water in a large pot and cook the lasagna noodles according to the package directions. Drain and rinse noodles with hot water, drizzle with 1 tbsp olive oil and gently stir to coat the noodles. Set aside. In a large skillet, heat 2 tablespoons olive oil over medium-high heat. Add the onion, eggplant, mushroom and red pepper. Cook the vegetables, stirring occasionally, until brown (15 minutes). Add 2 minced garlic cloves and cook for 30 seconds. Lower heat to medium, add tomatoes with their juice, 1 tsp salt, black pepper, red pepper flakes, dried basil and oregano and cook until most of the tomato liquid has reduced and the mixture is thick and cooked through. Preheat oven to 350 F. Place the soaked cashews in a blender with ⅓ cup water, the remaining

2 minced garlic cloves, lemon juice and nutritional yeast. Blend until smooth, scraping down the sides of the blender as needed. If needed, add more water, a little at a time. Remove half the mixture and reserve. To the remaining cashew cheese, add the fresh basil and remaining ¼ cup of olive oil and blend until smooth. Ladle a little of the liquid from the tomato vegetable mixture on the bottom of a 9×12 inch baking dish, then layer half the lasagna noodles. Add half of the tomato vegetable mixture and top with the basil cashew cheese. Layer on the remaining lasagna noodles, then the rest of the tomato vegetable mixture and drizzle the top with the reserved cashew cheese. Bake uncovered until hot and bubbly, 30-40 minutes.

WEEK 1 SATURDAY
....

Blueberry Hemp Smoothie (MAKES 2.5 CUPS)

2 tbsp hemp seeds

1 C fresh or frozen blueberries

½ C unsweetened almond, rice or hemp milk

½ C filtered water

1 tsp pure vanilla extract

½ tsp cinnamon

1 scoop protein powder (optional; ask your ND for a recommendation)

DIRECTIONS: Put all ingredients into blender or Magic Bullet and blend until smooth.

Crispy Breakfast Bars (16 BARS)

7 C crispy puffed rice whole-grain cereal

¾ C organic dried cranberries

¾ C organic dried blueberries

½ C sunflower seeds

1 tsp cinnamon

¾ C brown rice syrup or honey

¾ C almond butter

2 tbsp coconut oil

DIRECTIONS: Stir together cereal, dried fruits, seeds and cinnamon in large bowl. Place syrup, almond butter and coconut oil in a large pot. Melt on stove until butter substitute has melted. Stir well and pour over cereal mixture. Stir to coat. Dampen your hands with cold water. Press cereal mixture firmly into a 9-inch square baking pan, rewetting hands if necessary to keep mixture from sticking. Freeze 30 minutes. Cut into 16 bars and store in refrigerator.

Cranberry Quinoa Salad (SERVES 6)

2 C cooked quinoa
½ C hemp seeds
1 C chopped parsley
1 coarsely grated carrot
3 tbsp pumpkin seeds
3 tbsp dried cranberries

DRESSING
2 tsp hemp seed oil
2 tbsp lemon juice
1 tsp raw honey
½ tsp grey sea salt or pink rock salt

DIRECTIONS: Combine all salad ingredients in a large bowl. Combine all dressing ingredients in a small glass jar with a tight-fitting lid, and shake well. Toss the salad and dressing and serve immediately.

Shrimp in Thai Green Curry (SERVES 4)

1 tbsp coconut oil
2–3 cloves garlic, sliced thinly
10-15 baby asparagus spears
1 12-oz can coconut milk (not light)
1 tbsp Thai Kitchen Green Curry Paste
½ tsp turmeric
½ tsp red pepper flakes
1 lb shrimp, fresh or frozen and defrosted
½ tsp Thai Kitchen Fish Sauce (optional)
¼ C fresh basil leaves

DIRECTIONS: Heat the oil in a deep skillet over high heat and, when hot, sauté the garlic and asparagus until a little soft. Slowly pour the coconut milk into the skillet, and then add the Thai Kitchen Green Curry Paste, turmeric and red pepper flakes. Using a spatula, thoroughly mix the paste into the coconut milk, while bringing it to a light boil. Add the shrimp and fish sauce, if using. Cover the skillet (use aluminum foil if you don't have a lid), turn the heat down to medium, and cook for 10 minutes, stirring occasionally. Add the basil leaves and cook for about 1 minute more. Serve with wild rice, either plain or see recipe below.

Wild Rice (SERVES 4)

1 C wild rice
1 C organic vegetable broth
2 C water
2 stalks celery, diced
4 oz water chestnuts, diced
2 to 3 tbsp organic raisins

DIRECTIONS: Rinse the rice in a strainer and transfer it to a pot. Add the broth and water. Bring this to a boil over high heat, then cover and reduce heat to simmer. After 20 minutes, add the celery, water chestnuts and raisins to the rice and stir. The rice should be fully cooked in 40-50 minutes. Fluff it with a fork and drain off any excess water.

WEEK 1 SUNDAY

....

Breakfast Sausages (MAKES 9)

1 lb ground turkey
1 egg, lightly beaten (optional)
1 tsp ground sea salt
½ tsp ground sage
⅛ tsp ground nutmeg
⅛ tsp ground ginger

¼ tsp black pepper

3 shakes cayenne pepper

2 shakes dried thyme

1 ½ tsp organic olive oil

¾ tsp honey

DIRECTIONS: Place ground turkey in a large bowl, add egg and mix well. Combine salt and seasonings. Sprinkle the seasonings over the meat and work in until the seasonings are evenly distributed. Spread the olive oil over the meat and work in. Drizzle honey over the meat and work in. Shape into nine patties and fry at medium heat. Cover in between turnings. Turn frequently and watch closely. Cook for approximately 10-15 minutes.

Garden Bean Soup (SERVES 8)

1 tsp olive oil

2 chopped onions

1 C diced carrots

1 C chopped celery

2 tsp grated fresh ginger

1 tsp minced garlic

1 tsp garam masala (available at an Indian grocery store)

1 tsp turmeric

½ tsp ground cumin

½ tsp cayenne pepper

6 C organic vegetable broth

1 C lentils, uncooked

2 15-oz cans garbanzo beans, rinsed and drained

1 14.5-oz can diced tomatoes, undrained

DIRECTIONS: Pour olive oil into a large soup pot set over medium-high heat and sauté onions 3 to 4 minutes or until tender. Add carrots and celery and cook for 5 minutes. Stir in garlic and next four ingredients and cook for 30 seconds. Add broth and remaining ingredients and cook until lentils are tender, about 90 minutes. If desired, half of the soup can be pureed and stirred back into the pot for a thicker, creamier soup.

Lentil Dip (MAKES 3 CUPS)

1 16-oz can, drained, or 2 C cooked lentil
1 C almond butter or chopped walnuts
2 tbsp hemp seed oil
1 large clove garlic
½ C fresh basil OR 2 tbsp dairy- and nut-free basil pesto
⅓ C lemon juice
1 tsp lemon zest
1 tsp turmeric
¼ tsp grey sea salt or pink rock salt

DIRECTIONS: Process all ingredients in a food processor fitted with the S-blade until very smooth.

Almond Chicken (SERVES 2)

½ C ground almonds
1 tbsp dried oregano
1 tbsp dried basil
1 tbsp dried parsley
½ tsp sea salt
1 tsp freshly ground pepper
2 tbsp extra virgin olive oil
2 boneless, skinless chicken breasts

DIRECTIONS: Preheat oven to 450 F. Combine the almonds, oregano, basil, parsley, salt and pepper in a small bowl. Rinse the chicken breasts and pat dry with paper towel and place on a plate. Gently pat the chicken on each side with the almond mixture and place on a baking sheet or in a shallow glass baking dish. Drizzle the olive oil over the chicken and bake in the oven for 12 to 15 minutes, depending on the thickness of each breast.

Asian Asparagus (SERVES 2 TO 4)

1 bunch asparagus
½ C water
1 tbsp sesame oil
1 tsp sunflower oil

1 tsp freshly ground pepper

½ tsp sea salt

2 tbsp sesame seeds

DIRECTIONS: Wash asparagus, break off the hard ends. Put the asparagus and water in a large sauté pan and place on the stove over medium-high heat. Cover and steam for 3 minutes. Uncover, reduce the heat to low and add the sesame and sunflower oils, salt, pepper and sesame seeds. Stir to coat and cook, uncovered, for another 5 minutes.

WEEK 2 MONDAY

Grain-Free Berry Muffins (YIELDS 12 MUFFINS)

2 ½ C almond flour

1 tsp baking soda

½ tsp sea salt

1 tbsp cinnamon

½ C organic extra virgin olive oil

3 large organic eggs

½ C unpasteurized liquid honey

1 tbsp pure vanilla extract

1 C organic blueberries or raspberries, fresh or frozen

DIRECTIONS: Preheat oven to 300 F. Line a standard 12-cup muffin tin with paper liners. In a medium bowl, whisk together the almond flour, baking soda, salt and cinnamon. Add the oil, eggs, honey and vanilla to the dry ingredients and stir until the batter is smooth. Gently fold in the blueberries just until they are evenly distributed throughout the batter. Divide the batter between muffin cups. Bake on the centre rack for 35 minutes, rotating the pan after 15 minutes. A toothpick inserted into the centre of the muffin should come out clean. Let the muffins stand for 15 minutes, then transfer to a wire rack and let cool completely. Store the muffins in an airtight container at room temperature for up to 3 days.

Trail Mix (MAKES ¾ CUP)

4 oz raw unsalted pumpkin seeds
4 oz raw unsalted sunflower seeds
4 oz raisins

DIRECTIONS: Combine and store in a container in the refrigerator to avoid rancidity if storing for long periods of time.

This trail mix recipe is very high in iron and other essential nutrients. Use to replace unhealthy sugar-based sweets and chocolate for a snack food. It is a great mix to take on trips and can also be eaten for breakfast.

Ginger Butternut Soup (SERVES 6)

2 C finely chopped onions
1 tbsp extra virgin olive oil (organic)
2 cloves garlic, minced
10 C (2.5 L) filtered water or vegetable stock
7 C (1.75 L) butternut squash, peeled and diced
1 C red split lentils
1 tbsp minced fresh ginger root OR ½ teaspoon powdered ginger root
1 tsp ground cinnamon
¼ tsp ground nutmeg
3 tbsp tahini
1 tsp sea salt
parsley, watercress (optional)

DIRECTIONS: In a large soup pot over medium-low heat, cook the onion in the oil about 2 to 3 minutes, until the onions are translucent. Stir in the garlic, and then add the water or stock. Add squash and lentils. Cover and bring to a boil over high heat. Uncover pot and skim off lentil foam with a spoon. Reduce heat and simmer until the squash and lentils are tender, about 40 minutes. Using a blender, food processor or immersion blender, puree the squash mixture along with the spices, tahini and salt. Serve hot, garnished with roasted pumpkin or squash seeds and parsley or watercress, if desired.

Hummus
See Week 1 Wednesday.

Flax Baked Chicken (SERVES 2)

2 tbsp brown rice flour
1 tbsp ground flaxseed
1 tsp dried parsley
1 tsp dried paprika
1 tsp garlic powder
½ tsp turmeric
½ tsp sea salt
1 tsp freshly ground pepper
2 boneless, skinless chicken breasts
3 tbsp organic extra virgin olive oil

DIRECTIONS: Preheat oven to 450 F. In a small mixing bowl, combine the flour, flaxseed, parsley, paprika, garlic powder, turmeric, salt and pepper. Place the flour mixture in a zipper bag. Rinse and pat the chicken breasts dry. Coat the breasts with olive oil. Put the chicken in the bag with the flour mixture and thoroughly coat each piece. Place the chicken on a baking sheet or shallow glass baking dish and bake for 12 to 15 minutes, depending on the thickness of the chicken.

Roasted Beets and Spinach Salad (SERVES 2)

6 small beets, boiled and quartered
1 fennel bulb, tops cut off and bulb quartered
2 tbsp plus ¼ C extra virgin olive oil
4 C loosely packed baby spinach leaves
1 small avocado, peeled and diced
1 small shallot, minced
juice of half a lemon
½ tsp sea salt
½ tsp freshly ground pepper
½ C walnut halves, toasted

DIRECTIONS: Preheat oven to 450 F. Place the beets and fennel on a baking sheet, drizzle the 2 tablespoons of olive oil over top, and roast in the oven for 15 minutes. Meanwhile, combine the spinach and avocado in a mixing bowl. To make the dressing, put the shallot, lemon juice, salt, pepper and the ¼ cup of olive oil in a small food processor and pulse for 1 minute. Toss the dressing with the spinach and avocado and place on two serving plates. Place half the roasted beets and fennel on each plate and sprinkle the walnuts over each serving.

WEEK 2 TUESDAY
....

Warm Quinoa Porridge (SERVES 2)

2 C filtered water
¾ rolled quinoa flakes
1 tsp cinnamon
½ tsp cardamom powder
¼ tsp nutmeg
¼ tsp turmeric
1 tbsp raw honey
1/8 tsp sea salt
½ C organic apple, diced
½ C organic blueberries (if frozen, add before quinoa to thaw)
¼ C chopped almonds or hemp seeds

DIRECTIONS: Boil water in a small saucepan. Add the rolled quinoa and stir for 2 to 3 minutes. Remove from heat and mix in spices, raw honey, apple, blueberries and almonds.

Wonderful Whatever Salad (SERVES 1)

any green leafy lettuce (not iceberg) or spinach
cucumber
scallion, diced
tomato or bell peppers
sliced almonds
artichoke hearts (packed in water, not oil)
hemp nut seeds
Flax Baked Chicken, left over from night before

DIRECTIONS: Prepare the ingredients in the desired amounts and toss with any dressing!

Vegetarian Chili (serve with Avocado Salsa) (SERVES 6)

2 tsp canola oil

1 C chopped onion

1 C chopped red bell pepper

2 tsp chili powder

1 tsp ground cumin

1 tsp dried oregano

3 cloves garlic, minced

1 4.5-oz can chopped green chilies

⅔ C uncooked quick-cooking barley

¼ C water

1 15-oz can diced tomatoes, undrained

2 C vegetable broth

3 tbsp chopped fresh cilantro

6 lime wedges

18 baked organic tortilla chips

DIRECTIONS: Heat oil over medium-high heat. Add onion and bell pepper; sauté 3 minutes. Add chili powder and next 4 ingredients (chili powder through green chilies); cook 1 minute. Stir in barley and next 4 ingredients (barley through broth); bring to a boil. Cover, reduce heat, and simmer for 20 minutes or until barley is tender. Stir in cilantro. Serve with lime wedges, chips and Avocado Salsa.

Avocado Salsa (MAKES 1 CUP)

½ C finely chopped avocado

⅓ C chopped seeded tomato

2 tbsp finely chopped onion

1 tbsp finely diced seeded jalapeno pepper

1 tbsp chopped fresh cilantro

1 tbsp fresh lime juice

⅛ tsp salt

DIRECTIONS: Combine all ingredients; toss.

WEEK 2 WEDNESDAY

....

Berry-Almond Slam Smoothie (SERVES 1)

1½ C frozen mixed berries (strawberries, blueberries, and raspberries)
1½ C almond milk
1 tbsp almond butter
1 serving protein powder

DIRECTIONS: Put all ingredients in a food processor or blender and pulse until smooth, adding more liquid if necessary.

Warm Spicy Sweet Potato Salad (SERVES 4)

2 medium sweet potatoes, diced
1 small red onion, diced
1 tbsp plus ¼ C extra virgin olive oil
1 C loosely packed, chopped fresh cilantro
1 can adzuki beans, drained and rinsed
1 yellow bell pepper, seeded and diced
1 clove garlic, coarsely chopped
1 jalapeno pepper seeded
juice of 1 lime
½ tsp sea salt
½ tsp freshly ground pepper

DIRECTIONS: Preheat oven to 450 F. Place the sweet potatoes and onion on a baking sheet and drizzle with the 1 tablespoon of olive oil to coat. Roast in oven for 25 minutes. While the sweet potatoes are roasting, toss the cilantro, beans, and the bell pepper in a small bowl. To make the dressing, combine the garlic, jalapeno pepper, lime, salt and pepper in a small food chopper or processor. Process for 10 seconds and then add ¼ cup of olive oil and continue to process for another minute. Toss the roasted sweet potatoes and onion with the bean mixture and pour the dressing over top. Combine to thoroughly coat and serve warm.

Krispy Kale Chips
See Week 1 Thursday.

Sesame-Seed-Crusted Salmon Burgers (SERVES 4)

1 x 1-lb wild salmon fillet, skinned and chopped

2 C chopped baby spinach

¼ C panko (Japanese breadcrumbs)

1 tbsp fresh lemon juice, divided

1 tbsp tamari

¼ C sesame seeds, toasted and divided

¼ tsp salt

¼ tsp black pepper

olive oil cooking spray

DIRECTIONS: Combine salmon, spinach, panko, lemon juice, ginger, soy sauce, 1 tablespoon sesame seeds, sal and pepper in a large bowl. Form mixture into 4 (3½ -inch) patties. Place remaining sesame seeds onto a plate, and dip one side of patties into seeds to coat. Preheat a lightly oiled grill pan over medium heat until hot but not smoking. Cook burgers over medium heat, turning, 3-4 minutes per side or until golden brown and cooked through.

Chickpea Slaw (SERVES 4)

2 medium carrots, peeled and shredded

1 small bunch of kale, shredded

½ small head of red cabbage, shredded

1 19-oz can chickpeas, drained and rinsed

2 tbsp pumpkin seeds

1 tsp dried dill OR 1 tbsp snipped fresh dill

1 tsp dried oregano OR 1 tbsp chopped fresh organic oregano

½ tsp sea salt

½ tsp freshly ground pepper

½ tsp chili pepper flakes

½ C organic extra virgin olive oil

juice of 1 lemon

DIRECTIONS: Mix the carrots, kale, cabbage, chickpeas and pumpkin seeds in a serving bowl and set aside. To make the dressing, combine the dill, oregano, salt, chili pepper flakes and pepper in a small bowl, and then add the olive oil and lemon juice and whisk until well blended. Pour the dressing over the slaw, tossing to coat evenly.

WEEK 2 THURSDAY

....

Blueberry Buckwheat Pancakes

See Week 1 Wednesday.

Edamame and Bean Salad with Shrimp and Fresh Salsa

(SERVES 4)

EDAMAME AND BEAN SALAD

¼ C frozen shelled edamame

½ C chopped cooked small shrimp (about 3 oz)

½ C canned cannellini beans, rinsed and drained

½ C halved cherry tomatoes

1 to 2 tbsp chopped red onion

1 tsp minced jalapeno pepper

1 tbsp chopped fresh cilantro

2 tsp fresh lime juice

1 ½ tsp organic extra virgin olive oil

⅛ tsp salt

DIRECTIONS: Cook edamame according to package directions. Drain and rinse with cold water. Combine edamame, shrimp, cannellini beans, cherry tomatoes, onion and jalapeno pepper. Combine cilantro and the remaining ingredients, stirring with a whisk. Drizzle over edamame mixture, and toss gently to combine. Cover and chill.

Spaghetti Squash and Black Bean Tacos (SERVES 4)

1 to 2 lb spaghetti squash (if you go bigger, increase spices accordingly)

juice of 1 lime (about 2 tbsp)

1 tsp chili powder

1 tsp sea salt

1 tsp garlic powder

1 14-oz can black beans, thoroughly rinsed

8 to 10 crispy organic corn tacos

cilantro

hot sauce (optional)

DIRECTIONS: Preheat oven to 400 F. Cut spaghetti squash in half lengthwise, scoop out the seeds, spread 1 teaspoon olive oil on each half, and roast both halves face down on a rimmed baking sheet until tender and easily pierced with a fork, 45–60 minutes. Meanwhile, combine lime juice, chili powder, salt, and garlic powder in a small bowl. When spaghetti squash is done, remove from oven and let cool until you can handle it easily. Working over a large bowl, gently scrape out the flesh with a fork. Add lime mixture to the squash and toss well to combine. In the bottom of each corn taco, spread 2 table-spoons of black beans. Top with spaghetti squash. Line the tacos in a 9×13″ baking dish and bake in preheated oven for 20 minutes. To serve, top with fresh cilantro and hot sauce if desired.

WEEK 2 FRIDAY

Instant Flax Seed Cereal (SERVES 1)

6 tbsp raw flax seeds
4 to 8 oz non-dairy milk (soy, almond, rice)
½ banana, sliced

DIRECTIONS: Grind flax seeds to a powder using a coffee or seed grinder. Place powder in a cereal bowl and slowly add non-dairy milk, stirring the mixture together. The flax mixture will thicken into a cereal with a texture similar to cream of rice or oatmeal. Top cereal with sliced bananas. Eat the mixture right away because the flax seeds are sensitive to light, air and temperature. Eat it cold. Do not cook this cereal.

Trail Mix
See Week 2 Monday.

Fresh Salad Rolls (SERVES 4)

8 leaves of Boston or Bibb lettuce
2 carrots, peeled and julienned
½ cucumber, peeled and julienned

3 green onions, thinly sliced, white and pale green parts only

1 C loosely packed, chopped fresh cilantro

1 C loosely packed, chopped fresh mint

1 C finely chopped almonds

½ package thin rice vermicelli noodles or bean thread noodles, cooked

8 Vietnamese rice paper wrappers

DIRECTIONS: The easiest way to put together the salad rolls is to make an assembly line on the kitchen countertop or table, starting with the lettuce leaves. Fill a large bowl with warm water. Submerge 1 rice paper wrapper in the water for 10 seconds, or just until it becomes soft. Remove the wrapper to a flat work surface, and let it rest for 30 seconds; it will become easier to handle.

Place 1 leaf of lettuce just below the middle of the wrapper, leaving a 1-inch border on each side. Top with ¼ cup of the noodles, then 2 or 3 slices of the cucumber and carrots. Sprinkle a few green onions and cilantro and mint on the veggies, then top with some of the almonds.

Fold the bottom of the wrapper up over the filling, pressing the filling as you go. Fold both sides of the wrapper inward. Gently press to seal and roll the wrapper to the top edge. Repeat with the remaining wrappers.

Tangy Almond Dipping Sauce

1 piece of fresh gingerroot, chopped

1 clove garlic, chopped

2 tablespoons almond butter

juice of 1 lime

1 tsp chili pepper flakes

1½ tbsp sesame oil

½ C water, or more if a water consistency is more desired

¼ tsp sea salt

DIRECTIONS: In a food processor or blender, mince the gingerroot and garlic. Add the almond butter, lime juice, and chili pepper flakes and blend. Lastly, add the sesame oil, water, and salt and blend until smooth.

Lentil Dip
See Week 1 Sunday.

Almond Chicken
See Week 1 Sunday.

Stewed Kale and Lentils (SERVES 4)

1 tbsp organic extra virgin olive oil
1 red onion
3 cloves garlic, minced
1 tbsp minced fresh ginger
1 carrot, peeled and diced
1 tsp ground cumin
½ tsp ground cumin
½ tsp cinnamon
1 C dried green lentils
3 C organic vegetable broth
4 C chopped, stemmed kale
¼ C golden raisins
¼ C chopped walnuts, toasted

DIRECTIONS: In oven, heat oil over medium heat; cook onion, garlic and ginger, stirring occasionally, until softened, about 5 minutes. Add carrot, cumin and cinnamon; cook, stirring occasionally, until fragrant, about 3 minutes. Stir in lentils to coat. Add broth and bring to boil; reduce heat, cover and simmer until lentils are al dente, about 10 minutes. Add kale and raisins; simmer, covered, until lentils are tender, about 10 minutes. Uncover and cook until almost no liquid remains, about 4 minutes. Sprinkle with toasted walnuts.

Warm Oat and Apple Bowl (SERVES 1)

2 tbsp organic olive oil or organic coconut oil
2 tbsp steel-cut oats
1 tbsp organic apple puree (no sugar added)
2 tsp flaked almonds
2 tsp pumpkin seeds
2 tsp ground, raw almonds

DIRECTIONS: Heat the oil gently in a small saucepan. Add the oats and stir until starting to go golden. Add rest of ingredients and stir until starting to go golden. Add rest of ingredients and stir until heated through. Put in a bowl.

Arugula Rainbow Salad (SERVES 2)

2 C arugula, torn into large pieces
1½ C broccoli florets
1 C coarsely grated carrot
½ C finely diced radish
1 tbsp minced red onion
3 oz cooked chicken breast (optional)

DIRECTIONS: Place arugula, broccoli, carrot, radish and onion in a medium bowl. Top with dressing of choice. Add chicken if including.

Trail Mix
See Week 2 Monday.

Ultimate Turkey and Spinach Lasagna (MAKES 9 SERVINGS)

1 tbsp olive oil
1 medium onion, chopped (2 C)
2 cloves garlic, minced
¾ lb ground free-range turkey breast

3 C low-sodium organic marinara sauce

1.5 C organic, vegan ricotta cheese

1 10-oz package frozen spinach, completely defrosted
and squeezed of all excess liquid

¼ C chopped parsley

2 egg whites

¼ tsp salt

¼ tsp pepper

12 lasagna noodles, cooked al dente according to the package instructions

½ C shredded organic vegan mozzarella-like cheese

DIRECTIONS: Preheat oven to 375 F. Heat oil in a large, high-sided skillet and cook onion, stirring occasionally, until softened, 6-7 minutes. Add garlic and cook 1 minute. Add turkey and cook, breaking up with a spoon, until no longer pink and cooked through, 4–5 minutes. Add marinara, bring to a boil, reduce heat, and simmer 2–3 minutes. Remove pan from heat and cool slightly. Combine ricotta, spinach, parsley, egg whites, sal and pepper in a large bowl. Coat the bottom of a 14 × 11" lasagna pan with ½ cup sauce, arrange three lasagna noodles on the bottom of the pan. Spread ¾ cup sauce evenly over noodles. Spoon ⅔ cup ricotta-spinach mixture evenly on top of sauce. Repeat layers two more times. Cover top with three noodles and remaining ¾ cup sauce. Sprinkle the mozzarella and parmesan. Cover loosely with foil and bake for 45 minutes. Remove foil and bake 10-15 minutes, until cheese is bubbly. Cut into 9 squares and serve.

WEEK 2 SUNDAY
....

Rice Bread with Sliced Avocado (SERVES 1)

rice bread, 1 slice
avocado (half)

DIRECTIONS: Place one piece of rice bread in the toaster. Slice half of an avocado lengthwise and place on top of toast. Can also mash half an avocado onto the toast.

Garden Bean Soup

See Week 1 Sunday.

Pumpkin-Seed-Crusted Halibut (SERVES 2)

½ tbsp coriander
¼ C chopped raw pumpkin seeds
¼ C olive oil
1 lb halibut fillet, cut into two pieces
3 tbsp butter
1 lemon
1 tbsp chopped parsley

DIRECTIONS: Preheat oven to 350 F. Add the coriander to the pumpkin seeds, and then chop the seeds in a food processor, being careful to avoid flourlike texture. Meanwhile, spread the olive oil over the bottom of a baking dish. Dredge the halibut through the olive oil so that all sides of the fish are lightly coated. With one hand, spoon the chopped pumpkin seeds onto all sides of the fish, while using the fingers of your other hand to pat the seeds onto the fish. Add 1½ tablespoons butter to the top of each piece of fish. Bake the fish 10 minutes per inch of thickness. When it's done, squeeze lemon juice on each piece of fish and sprinkle with parsley.

Kale Salad (SERVES 4)

6 C kale, chopped
½ lemon
pinch dried basil
pinch grey sea salt or pink rock salt
1 tbsp extra virgin olive, camelina, flax or hemp seed oil
2 tbsp red onion, minced
2 tbsp green onion, chopped (about 1 whole onion)
1 small cucumber, thinly sliced
1 clove garlic, minced
¼ C chopped Kalamata olives

DIRECTIONS: Wash kale and cut into small strips. Steam for 5–7 minutes and transfer to bowl and add lemon, basil, salt and oil. Toss. Add the remaining ingredients and mix well.

Acknowledgements

AS WITH MOST health conditions, the boundaries of disease extend beyond the individual who is suffering. Mental illness is no exception. There are many people to thank. Over the years, I have been counselled, supported, cared for and loved by so many. The list below is not exhaustive, and I owe gratitude to many who aren't listed below.

Thank you to my family members, both living and deceased, who have stood by me through thick and thin. I bow my head in grace to you.

Thank you to my dear, sweet, amazing friends: Lisa, Tracey, Cheryl, Pearl, Debra, Colleen, Barb, Gareth and many more.

Thank you to my husband's family—I know it hasn't been easy to know me from a distance, and I thank you for making the effort.

Thank you to my many colleagues who have shaped my knowledge, guided my experience and supported my growth. Most notably: Dr. Larry Chan, Dr. Jason Hughes and Dr. Orna Villazan.

Thank you to Dr. Ron Remick for being an amazing psychiatrist to me for 20 years.

Thank you to Dr. Abram Hoffer for starting me on the orthomolecular path to health. Thank you to Dr. Jonathon Prousky for stepping into Dr. Hoffer's shoes and carrying on the important message of orthomolecular and naturopathic healthcare.

Thank you to Steven Carter and Andrew Cuscianna for giving me a platform to share my story and believing in me.

Thank you to all my patients and staff. I am blessed to walk the path of health with each and every one of you. You are as much my guide as I am yours.

Thank you to all who had a hand in the creation of this book. To my editor, Patti Ryan, I remain in awe of your brilliance, humour and skill. To the team at PageTwo Strategies, thank you for all your help and encouragement.

Lastly, thank you to my husband and my son. I didn't know I could love so much and that I would be capable of receiving so much love from each of you. I love you both with all my heart.

Bibliography & Recommended Reading

A Course in Miracles. Penguin Arkana, 1975.

Aggarwal, Ameet. *Heal Your Body: Cure Your Mind.* CreateSpace, 2013.

Aron, Elaine. *The Highly Sensitive Person: How to Thrive When the World Overwhelms You.* Broadway Books, 1996.

Bernstein, Gabrielle. *May Cause Miracles.* Harmony Books, 2013.

Bongiorno, Peter. *Healing Depression.* CCNM Press, 2010.

Bolte-Taylor, Jill. *My Stroke of Insight.* Penguin Group, 2008.

Brach, Tara. *Radical Self-Acceptance.* Bantam Books, 2003.

Breathnach, Sarah Ban. *Something More.* Time Warner International, 2000.

Brown, Brené. *The Gifts of Imperfection.* Hazelden, 2010.

Cameron, Julia. *The Artist's Way.* Penguin Putnam, 1995.

Chodron, Pema. *Living Beautifully with Uncertainty and Change.* Shambhala Publications, 2012

Chodron, Pema. *Start Where You Are.* Shambhala Publications, 2001.

Chodron, Pema. *Taking the Leap.* Shambhala Publications, 2009

Chodron, Pema. *When Things Fall Apart.* Shambhala Publications, 1997.

Chopra, Deepak. *Ageless Body, Timeless Mind.* Random House, 1993.

Chopra, Deepak; Ford, Debbie; Williamson, Marianne. *The Shadow Effect: Illuminating the Hidden Power of Your True Self.* HarperOne, 2010.

Coelho, Paulo. *The Alchemist.* HarperCollins, 1995.

Covey, Stephen. *The 7 Habits of Highly Effective People: Powerful Lessons in Personal Change.* Simon & Schuster, 1989.

Crinnion, Walter. *Clean, Green & Lean: Get Rid of the Toxins That Make You Fat.* John Wiley & Sons, 2010.

Doidge, Norman. *The Brain that Changes Itself.* Penguin Books, 2007.

Dweck, Carol. *Mindset: The New Psychology of Success.* Ballantine Books, 2006.

Dyer, Wayne. *Getting in the Gap.* Hay House, 2003.

Dyer, Wayne. *I Can See Clearly Now.* Hay House 2014.

Dyer, Wayne. *Wishes Fulfilled.* Hay House Inc., 2012

Ford, Debbie. *The Right Questions.* HarperCollins, 2003.

Frankl, Viktor. *Man's Search for Meaning.* Washington Square Press, 1984.

Gawain, Shakti. *Living in the Light.* Nataraj Publishing, 1986.

Gillson, George; Marsden, Tracy. *You've Hit Menopause Now What?*
    3 Simple Steps to Restoring Hormone Balance. Blitzprint, 2004.

Gibran, Kahil. *The Prophet.* Arrow, 2000.

Goleman, Daniel. *Emotional Intelligence.* Bantam Books, 1995.

Greenberger, Dennis; Padesky, Christine. *Mind over Mood.* The Guilford Press, 1995.

Hall, Karyn D. *The Emotionally Sensitive Person: Finding Peace When Your Emotions
    Overwhelm You,* New Harbinger Publications, 2014.

Hay, Louise. *The Power Is Within You.* Hay House, 1991.

Hay, Louise. *You Can Heal Your Life.* Hay House, 1984.

Hay, Louise; Richardson, Cheryl. *You Can Create An Exceptional Life.*
    Hay House, 2011.

Holden, Robert. *Be Happy!* Hay House, 2009.

Holden, Robert. *Loveability.* Hay House, 2013.

Holden, Robert. *Success Intelligence.* Hay House, 2005.

Jeffers, Susan. *Feel the Fear and Do It Anyways.* Rider, 1991.

Jensen, Karen; Schauch, Marita. *The Adrenal Stress Connection*
    Act Natural, 2010.

Kabat-Zinn, John. *Wherever You Go There You Are.* Hyperion, 1994.

Katie, Byron; Mitchell, Stephen. *Loving What Is.* Harmony Books, 2002.

Levin, Nancy. *Jump! And Your Life Will Appear.* Hay House, 2014.

Lipton, Bruce. *The Biology of Belief.* Mountain of Love, 2005.

Maté, Gabor. *In the Realm of Hungry Ghosts: Close Encounters with Addiction.*
    Knopf Canada, 2008.

Maté, Gabor. *When the Body Says No: The Cost of Hidden Stress.* Knopf Canada, 2004.

McGonigal, Kelly. *The Willpower Instinct.* Penguin Group, 2012.

McLaren, Karla. *The Language of Emotions.* Sounds True, 2010.

Moorjani, Anita. *Dying to Be Me.* Hay House, 2012.

Murray, Michael; Pizzorno, Joseph. *Encyclopedia of Natural Medicine.*
    Prima Health, 1998.

Neufeld, Gordon; Maté, Gabor. *Hold On to Your Kids: Why Parents Need to Matter More
    Than Peers.* Ballantine Books, 2004.

Northrup, Christianne. *Mother-Daughter Wisdom.* Bantam Books, 2005.

Northrup, Christianne. *Women's Bodies, Women's Wisdom.* Bantam Books, 1994.

Peck, M. Scott. *The Road Less Travelled.* Touchstone, 1978.

Peterson, Christopher. *A Primer in Positive Psychology.* Oxford University Press, 2006.

Pollan, Michael. *In Defense of Food: An Eater's Manifesto.* Penguin Books, 2008.

Richardson, Cheryl. *Stand Up for Your Life*. Simon & Schuster, 2002.

Richardson, Cheryl. *Take Time for Your Life*. Broadway Books, 1999.

Richardson, Cheryl. *The Art of Extreme Self-Care*. Hay House, 2009.

Richardson, Cheryl. *The Unmistakable Touch of Grace*. Simon & Schuster. 2005.

Roth, Geneen. *Breaking Free From Compulsive Eating*. Plume, 2004

Roth, Geneen. *When Food Is Love*. Plume, 1991.

Roth, Geneen. *Women, Food and God*. Simon & Schuster, 2011.

Ruiz, Don Miguel. *The Four Agreements*. Amber-Allen Publishing, 1997

Ruiz, Don Miguel; Ruiz, Don Jose. *The Fifth Agreement*. Amber-Allen Publishing, 2011.

Sapolsky, Robert. *Why Zebras Don't Get Ulcers*. Henry Hold and Company, 1994.

Seligman, Martin. *Authentic Happiness*. Atria Paperback, 2002.

Seligman, Martin. *Flourish*. Free Press, 2011.

Selye, Hans. *The Stress of Life*. McGraw Hill, 1956.

Smith, Rick; Lourie, Bruce. *Slow Death by Rubber Duck*. Vintage Canada, 2009.

Tipping, Colin. *Radical Forgiveness*. Sounds True, 2009.

Tolle, Eckhart. *The Power of Now*. New World Library and Namaste Publishing, 1999.

Tolle, Eckhart. *A New Earth*. Penguin Books, 2005.

Walsch, Neale. *The Little Soul and the Sun*. Hampton Roads Publishing Company, 1998.

Williamson, Marianne. *A Return to Love*. HarperOne, 1996.

References

CHAPTER 1

Maté, G. (2008). *In the realm of hungry ghosts: Close encounters with addiction.* Toronto, ON: Knopf Canada.

Pizzorno, J. E., & Murray, M. (1999). *Textbook of natural medicine.* Edinburgh: Churchill Livingstone.

CHAPTER 2

American Psychiatric Association. (2013). *Diagnostic and statistical manual of mental disorders* (5th ed.). Washington, DC: Author.

Stoffstall, V. (1971). Comes the dawn. Publisher unknown.

CHAPTER 3

Mood Disorders Society of Canada. (2009, January). Quick facts: Mental illness and addictions in Canada. Retrieved from https://mdsc.ca/docs/Quick%20 Facts_3rd_Edition_Eng%20Nov_12_09.pdf.

CHAPTER 5

Santra, R., Chaudhuri, P. R., Dhali, D., & Mondal, S. (2012). Suicidality and suicide attempt in a young female on long-term sertraline treatment. *Indian Journal of Psychological Medicine, 34*(4), 391–393. doi:10.4103/0253-7176.108230

MedlinePlus Medical Encyclopedia. (2015). Antifreeze poisoning. Retrieved from https://medlineplus.gov/ency/article/002751.htm

Williamson, M. (1996). *A return to love: Reflections on the principles of a course in miracles.* San Francisco: HarperOne.

Greenblatt, J. (2015, April). [Presentation]. Presentation at the Mental Health Regained Public Forum. Toronto, ON.

Journal of Naturopathic Medicine

CHAPTER 8

http://orthomolecular.org/library/jom/1999/articles/1999-v14n01-p049.shtml

CHAPTER 10

Gillson, G., & Marsden, T. (2004). *You've hit menopause: Now what? 3 simple steps to restoring hormone balance.* Calgary: Blitzprint.

Neurotransmitter diagram: http://www.columbia.edu/cu/psychology/courses/1010/ mangels/neuro/transmission/transmission.gif

Essential. (2014). *Merriam-webster.com.* Retrieved May 8, 2014, from https://merriam-webster.com/dictionary/essential

Marz, R. B. (1999). *Medical nutrition from Marz: A textbook in clinical nutrition.* Portland, OR: Omni-Press.

DesMaisons, K. (2001). *Potatoes not Prozac: A natural seven-step dietary plan to control depression, food cravings and weight gain.* London: Pocket Books.

CHAPTER 11

Maes, M., Leonard, B. E., Myint, A. M., Kubera, M., & Verkerk, R. (2011). The new '5-HT' hypothesis of depression: Cell-mediated immune activation induces indoleamine 2,3-dioxygenase, which leads to lower plasma tryptophan and an increased synthesis of detrimental tryptophan catabolites (TRYCATs), both of which contribute to the onset of depression. *Progress in Neuro-Psychopharmacology & Biological Psychiatry, 35* (3): 702-721. doi:10.1016/ j.pnpbp.2010.12.017.PMID 21185346

CHAPTER 12

Sugar is a drug. (2012). *Hungry for Change.* Retrieved from http://www.hungryforchange.tv/article/sugar-is-a-drug

Chen, A. (2015). Is your caffeine addiction a preventative healthcare measure? *Dr. Alison Chen.* Retrieved from http://www.dralisonchen.com/2015/02/ is-your-caffeine-addiction-a-preventative-healthcare-measure/

Parry, N. (2015). Does caffeine affect the absorption of vitamins and minerals? *Livestrong.* Retrieved from http://www.livestrong.com/ article/464884-does-caffeine-affect-the-absorption-of-vitamins-or-minerals/

Robbins, C. (2017). Can drinking coffee cause diarrhea? *Livestrong.* Retrieved from http://www.livestrong.com/article/348718-can-drinking-coffee-cause-diarrhea/

Branch, S. (2014). Does coffee irritate stomach ulcers? *Livestrong.* Retrieved from http://www.livestrong.com/article/347548-does-coffee-irritate-stomach-ulcers/

Studies indicate lifestyle variations affect hypertension. *Today's Dietician.* Retrieved from http://www.todaysdietitian.com/news/070811_news.shtml

Katan, M., & Schouten, E. (2005). Caffeine and arrhythmia. *American Journal of Clinical Nutrition, 81,* 539-540.

Bond, O. (2015). How caffeine affects the nervous system. *Livestrong*. Retrieved from http://www.livestrong.com/ article/409740-how-caffeine-affects-the-nervous-system/

Fulghum Bruce, D. Chronic fatigue: Tired of feeling tired? *WebMD*. Retrieved from http://www.webmd.com/women/features/chronic-fatigue-tired-feeling-tired#1

Veracity, D. (2005). The hidden dangers of caffeine: How coffee causes exhaustion, fatigue, and addiction. *Natural News*. Retrieved from http://www.naturalnews.com/012352_caffeine_coffee.html

MacMahon, B., Yen, S., Trichopoulos, D., Warren, K., & Nardi, G. (1981). Coffee and cancer of the pancreas. *New England Journal of Medicine,*. 304(11), 630–633.

Mercola, J. (2009). Who knew preventing kidney stones was this easy? *Mercola*. Retrieved from http://articles.mercola.com/sites/articles/archive/2009/06/23/who-knew-preventing-kidney-stones-was-this-easy.aspx

Simpson, J. (2014). Which foods should you avoid with fibrocystic disease? *Livestrong*. Retrieved from http://www.livestrong.com/ article/327040-what-foods-should-you-avoid-with-fibrocystic-disease/

Caffeine content for coffee, tea, soda and more. (2014). *Mayo Clinic*. Retrieved from http://www.mayoclinic.org/healthy-lifestyle/nutrition-and-healthy-eating/ in-depth/caffeine/art-20049372

Cherney, K. (2015). What kind of coffee has the most caffeine? *Livestrong*. Retrieved from http://www.livestrong.com/ article/144174-what-kind-coffee-has-most-caffeine/

Derrer, D. T. (2014). Guarana. *WebMD*. Retrieved from http://www.webmd.com/diet/supplement-guide-guarana#2

Kola Nut. (2010). *Drugs-Forum*. Retrieved from https://drugs-forum.com/threads/kola-nut-cola-spp.116270/

Yerba maté tea. (n.d.) *Caffeine Informer*. Retrieved from https://www.caffeineinformer.com/caffeine-content/yerba-mate

CHAPTER 13

Foster, J., & McVey Neufeld, K.A. (2013). Gut-brain axis: How the microbiome influences anxiety and depression. *Trends in Neuroscience, 36*(5), 305–312. doi: 10.1016/j.tins.2013.01.005

Logan, A. C., & Katzman, M. (2005). Major depressive disorders: probiotics may be an adjuvant therapy. *Medical Hypothesis, 64*(3), 533–538.

People less focused on recurrent bad feelings when taking probiotics. (2015). *Science Daily*. Retrieved from https://www.sciencedaily.com/releases/2015/04/150414083718.htm

Aggarwal, A. (2016, February 13). How your liver affects your mind, mood, hormones, anxiety, stress and depression. [YouTube]. Retrieved from https://www.youtube.com/watch?v=BhF9feMjT3c

IgG food sensitivity. (n.d). *Rocky Mountain Analytical.* Retrieved from http://rmalab. com/medical-laboratory-tests/allergy/igg-sensitivity

Pizzorno, J. E., & Murray, M. (1999). *Textbook of natural medicine.* Edinburgh: Churchhill Livingstone.

Zand, J., & LaValle, J. B. (1999). *Smart medicine for healthier living: A practical A-to-Z reference to natural and conventional treatments.* New York: Avery.

CHAPTER 14

Park, A. (2016). This is what happens to your brain on no sleep. *Time Health.* Retrieved from http://time.com/4282023/ this-is-what-happens-to-your-brain-on-no-sleep/

Musnick, D., & Mercola, J. (n.d.). *Conscious Living Centre.* Retrieved from http://www.consciouslivingcenter.com/article_16.html

Vgontzas, A. N. (2001). Chronic insomnia is associated with nyctohemeral activation of the hypothalamic-pituitary-adrenal axis: Clinical mplications. *Journal of Clinical Endocrinology & Metabolism, 86*(8), 3787-3794. doi:10.1210/jc.86.8.3787

Peri, C. (2014). 10 things to hate about sleep loss. *WebMD.* Retrieved from http://www.webmd.com/sleep-disorders/features/10-results-sleep-loss#3

Quick Facts on Mental Illness and Addictions in Canada (3rd edition). (2009). *Mood Disorders Society of Canada.* Retrieved from http://www.mooddisorderscanada.ca/ page/quick-facts

CHAPTER 15

Smetanin, P., Stiff, D., Briante, C., Adair, C.E., Ahmad, S., & Khan, M. (2011). The life and economic impact of major mental illnesses in Canada: 2011 to 2041. *RiskAnalytica,* on behalf of the Mental Health Commission of Canada 2011. Retrieved from http://stg.mentalhealthcommission.ca/English/system/files/ private/document/MHCC_Report_Base_Case_FINAL_ENG_0.pdf

Lim, K. L., Jacobs, P., Ohinmaa, A., Schopflocher, D., & Dewa, C.S.(2008). A new population-based measure of the burden of mental illness in Canada. *Chronic Diseases in Canada, 28:* 92-8.

Statistics: Health at a glance. (2013). Organisation for Economic Co-operation and Development (OECD). Retrieved from http:// www.oecd-ilibrary.org/sites/health_glance-2013-en/04/10/ g4-10-04.html?contentType=&itemId=/content/Chapter/health_glance-2013-41-en&containerItemId=/content/serial/19991312&accessItemIds=/ content/book/health_glance-2013-en&mimeType=text/ html&_csp_=2f6481becc176514dc3acbdcffc1daaa

Craft, L. L., & Landers, D. M. (1998). The effect of exercise on clinical depression and depression resulting from mental illness: A meta-analysis. *Journal of Sport and Exercise Psychology, 20,* 339-357.

Petruzzello, S. J., Landers, D. M., Hatfield, B. D., Kubitz, K. A., & Salazar, W. (1991). A meta-analysis on the anxiety-reducing effects of acute and chronic exercise. *Sports medicine, 11*(3), 143-182.

Den Heijer, A. E., Groen, Y., Tucha, L., Fuermaier, A. B., Koerts, J., Lange, K. W., & Tucha, O. (2017). Sweat it out? The effects of physical exercise on cognition and behaviour in children and adults with ADHD: A systematic literature review. *Journal of Neural Transmission,* 124(Suppl 1):3-26. doi: 10.1007/s00702-016-1593-7

Carter, T., Morres, I. D., Meade, O., & Callaghan, P. (2016). The effect of exercise on depressive symptoms in adolescents: A systematic review and meta-analysis. *Journal of the American Academy of Child & Adolescent Psychiatry.*

Kvam, S., Kleppe, C. L., Nordhus, I. H., & Hovland, A. (2016). Exercise as a treatment for depression: A meta-analysis. *Journal of affective disorders, 202,* 67-86.

Mead, G. E., Morley, W., Campbell, P., Greig, C. A., McMurdo, M., & Lawlor, D. A. (2009). *Exercise for depression.* London: The Cochrane Library.

Beebe, L. H., Tian, L., Morris, N., Goodwin, A., Allen, S. S., & Kuldau, J. (2005). Effects of exercise on mental and physical health parameters of persons with schizophrenia. *Issues in Mental Health Nursing, 26*(6), 661-676.

Abrantes, A. M., Strong, D. R., Cohn, A., Cameron, A. Y., Greenberg, B. D., Mancebo, M. C., & Brown, R. A. (2009). Acute changes in obsessions and compulsions following moderate-intensity aerobic exercise among patients with obsessive-compulsive disorder. *Journal of Anxiety Disorders, 23*(7), 923-927.

Callaghan, P. (2004). Exercise: A neglected intervention in mental health care? *Journal of Psychiatric and Mental Health Nursing, 11*(4), 476-483.

Souza de Sa Filho, A., Marcos de Souza Moura, A., Khede Lamego, M., Barbosa Ferreira Rocha, N., Paes, F., Cristina Oliveira, A., & Wegner, M. (2015). Potential therapeutic effects of physical exercise for bipolar disorder. *CNS & Neurological Disorders-Drug Targets (Formerly Current Drug Targets-CNS & Neurological Disorders), 14*(10), 1255-1259.

Martinsen, E. W., Hoffart, A., & Solberg, Ø. (1989). Comparing aerobic with nonaerobic forms of exercise in the treatment of clinical depression: A randomized trial. *Comprehensive Psychiatry, 30*(4), 324-331.

Stathopoulou, G., Powers, M. B., Berry, A. C., Smits, J. A., & Otto, M. W. (2006). Exercise interventions for mental health: A quantitative and qualitative review. *Clinical Psychology: Science and Practice, 13*(2), 179-193.

Stephens, T. (1988). Physical activity and mental health in the United States and Canada: Evidence from four population surveys. *Preventive Medicine, 17*(1), 35-47.

Barton, J., & Pretty, J. (2010). What is the best dose of nature and green exercise for improving mental health? A multi-study analysis. *Environmental Science & Technology, 44*(10), 3947-3955.

Mackay, G. J., & Neill, J. T. (2010). The effect of "green exercise" on state anxiety and the role of exercise duration, intensity, and greenness: A quasi-experimental study. *Psychology of Sport and Exercise, 11*(3), 238-245.

Pretty, J., Peacock, J., Sellens, M., & Griffin, M. (2005). The mental and physical health outcomes of green exercise. *International Journal of Environmental Health research*, 15(5), 319-337.

De Moor, M. H. M., Beem, A. L., Stubbe, J. H., Boomsma, D. I., & De Geus, E. J. C. (2006). Regular exercise, anxiety, depression and personality: A population-based study. *Preventive Medicine*, 42(4), 273-279.

Lisanne, F., Bolandzadeh, N., Nagamatsu, L. S., Hsu, C. L., Davis, J. C., Miran-Khan, K., & Liu-Ambrose, T. (2015). Aerobic exercise increases hippocampal volume in older women with probable mild cognitive impairment: A 6-month randomized controlled trial. *British Journal of sports Medicine*, 49(4), 248.

Querido, J. S., & Sheel, A. W. (2007). Regulation of cerebral blood flow during exercise. *Sports Medicine*, 37(9), 765-782.

Metcalfe, A. W. S., MacIntosh, B. J., Scavone, A., Ou, X., Korczak, D., & Goldstein, B. I. (2016). Effects of acute aerobic exercise on neural correlates of attention and inhibition in adolescents with bipolar disorder. *Translational Psychiatry*, 6(5), e814.

Wood, J. (2016, February 28). Hard exercise can boost brain chemicals sapped by depression. *PsychCentral*. Retrieved from http://psychcentral.com/news/2016/02/28/people-who-exercise-have-better-mental-fitness/99703.html

Olson, A. K., Eadie, B. D., Ernst, C., & Christie, B. R. (2006). Environmental enrichment and voluntary exercise massively increase neurogenesis in the adult hippocampus via dissociable pathways. *Hippocampus*, 16(3), 250-260.

Godman, H. (2014, April 9). Regular exercise changes the brain to improve memory, thinking skills. *Harvard Health Blog*. Retrieved from http://www.health.harvard.edu/blog/regular-exercise-changes-brain-improve-memory-thinking-skills-201404097110

Deslandes, A., Moraes, H., Ferreira, C., Veiga, H., Silveira, H., Mouta, R., & Laks, J. (2009). Exercise and mental health: Many reasons to move. *Neuropsychobiology*, 59(4), 191-198.

Sparks, A. (2015). Lena Dunham on exercise: "It ain't about the ass." *PsychCentral*. Retrieved from http://blogs.psychcentral.com/your-mind/2015/04/lena-dunham-on-exercise-it-aint-about-the-ass/

Kelso, T. (n.d.). The right way to lose fat: How to exercise. *Breaking Muscle*. Retrieved from https://breakingmuscle.com/fuel/the-right-way-to-lose-fat-what-to-eat

CHAPTER 16

Dirty Dozen. (2017). *Environmental Working Group*. Retrieved from https://www.ewg.org/foodnews/dirty_dozen_list.php

Products containing triclosan. (n.d.). *Beyond Pesticides*. Retrieved from http://www.beyondpesticides.org/programs/antibacterials/triclosan/products-containing-triclosan

Anton, S. D., Martin, C. K., Han, H., Coulon, S., Cefalu, W. T., Geiselman, P., & Williamson, D. A. (2010). Effects of stevia, aspartame, and sucrose on food intake, satiety, and postprandial glucose and insulin levels. *Appetite, 55*(1), 37-43.

Aune, D. (2012). Soft drinks, aspartame, and the risk of cancer and cardiovascular disease. *The American Journal of Clinical Nutrition, 96*(6), 1249-1251.

Bjarnadottir, A. (2017). 5 Reasons why Vitaminwater is a bad idea. *Authority Nutrition.* Retreived from https://authoritynutrition. com/5-reasons-why-vitaminwater-is-a-bad-idea/

Baan, R., Grosse, Y., Lauby-Secretan, B., El Ghissassi, F., Bouvard, V., Benbrahim-Tallaa, L., & Straif, K. (2011). Carcinogenicity of radiofrequency electromagnetic fields. *Lancet Oncology, 12*(7), 624-626.

Microwave Oven Radiation. *EM Watch.* Retrieved from http://emwatch.com/ microwave-oven-radiation/

Environmental Working Group 2013.http://www.ewg.org/research/ healthy-home-tips/tip-6-skip-non-stick-avoid-dangers-teflon

Fagherazzi, G., Vilier, A., Sartorelli, D. S., Lajous, M., Balkau, B., & Clavel-Chapelon, F. (2013). Consumption of artificially and sugar-sweetened beverages and incident type 2 diabetes in the Etude Epidémiologique auprès des femmes de la Mutuelle Générale de l'Education Nationale–European Prospective Investigation into Cancer and Nutrition cohort. *American Journal of Clinical Nutrition, 97*(3), 517-523.

Hardell, L., Carlberg, M., Soderqvist, F., & Hansson Mild, K. (2008). Meta-analysis of long-term mobile phone use and the association with brain tumours. *International Journal of Oncology, 32*(5), 1097-1104.

Hand, L. (2010). Plastics: Danger where we least expect it. *Harvard Health.* Retrieved from https://www.hsph.harvard.edu/news/magazine/winter10plastics/

The Nutrition Source Artifical Sweeteners. *Harvard Health.* Retrieved from https:// www.hsph.harvard.edu/nutritionsource/healthy-drinks/artificial-sweeteners/

Harvard Health Publications (2006). Microwaving food in plastic: Dangerous or not? *Harvard Medical School.* Retrieved from http://www.health.harvard.edu/ staying-healthy/microwaving-food-in-plastic-dangerous-or-not

Mortazavi, S. M. J., Habib, A., Ganj-Karimi, A. H., Samimi-Doost, R., Pour-Abedi, A., & Babaie, A. (2015). Alterations in TSH and thyroid hormones following mobile phone use. *Iranian Journal of Medical Sciences, 34*(4), 299-300.

Hamilton, J. (2011) Study: Most plastics leach hormone-like chemicals. *NPR.* Retrieved from http://www.npr.org/2011/03/02/134196209/ study-most-plastics-leach-hormone-like-chemicals

Safespace. Microwave Oven Dangers. Retrieved from https://www. safespaceprotection.com/news-and-info/microwave-oven-dangers/

Shwide-Slavin, C., Swift, C., & Ross, T. (2012). Nonnutritive sweeteners: Where are we today? *Diabetes Spectrum, 25*(2), 104-110.

Soto, A. M., & Sonnenschein, C. (2010). Environmental causes of cancer: Endocrine disruptors as carcinogens. *Nature Reviews Endocrinology, 6*(7), 363-370.

Wang, T., Li, M., Chen, B., Xu, M., Xu, Y., Huang, Y.,... & Liu, Y. (2011). Urinary bisphenol A (BPA) concentration associates with obesity and insulin resistance. *Journal of Clinical Endocrinology & Metabolism*, 97(2), E223-E227.

World Health Organization: Electromagetic fields and public health: Microwave ovens. http://www.who.int/peh-emf/publications/facts/info_microwaves/en/

Darbre, P. D., & Harvey, P. W. (2008). Paraben esters: Review of recent studies of endocrine toxicity, absorption, esterase and human exposure, and discussion of potential human health risks. *Journal of Applied Toxicology*, 28(5), 561-578.

Gannon, Megan. (2014). Triclosan, found in antibacterial soap and other products, causes cancer in mice. *Washington Post*. Nov 24, 2014. Retrieved from https://www.washingtonpost.com/national/health-science/triclosan-found-in-antibacterial-soap-and-other-products-causes-cancer-in-mice/2014/11/24/096b8ca4-70cc-11e4-ad12-3734c461eab6_story.html

Handa, O., Kokura, S., Adachi, S., Takagi, T., Naito, Y., Tanigawa, T.,... & Yoshikawa, T. (2006). Methylparaben potentiates UV-induced damage of skin keratinocytes. *Toxicology*, 227(1), 62-72.

Kobylewski, S., & Jacobson, M. F. (2010). *Food dyes: A rainbow of risks*. Washington, DC: Center for Science in the Public Interest.

Potera, C. (2010). Diet and nutrition: The artificial food dye blues. *Environmental Health Perspectives*, 118(10), A428.

Walia, Arjun. (2014). 10 Scientific studies proving GMOs can be harmful to human health. *Collective Evoluton*. 8 April 2015. http://www.collective-evolution.com/2014/04/08/10-scientific-studies-proving-gmos-can-be-harmful-to-human-health/

Westervelt, Amy. (2015). Phthalates are everywhere, and the health risks are worrying. How bad are they really? *The Guardian*. Feb 10, 2015. https://www.theguardian.com/lifeandstyle/2015/feb/10/phthalates-plastics-chemicals-research-analysis

Bernstein, L., Henderson, B. E., Hanisch, R., Sullivan-Halley, J., & Ross, R. K. (1994). Physical exercise and reduced risk of breast cancer in young women. *Journal of the National Cancer institute*, 86(18), 1403-1408. https://www.ncbi.nlm.nih.gov/pubmed/8072034

Better Health. (2016) Obesity and Hormones. Written in consultation with Hudson Institute of Medical Research. https://www.betterhealth.vic.gov.au/health/healthyliving/obesity-and-hormones

Brent, G. A. (2010). Environmental exposures and autoimmune thyroid disease. *Thyroid*, 20(7), 755-761. https://www.ncbi.nlm.nih.gov/pmc/articles/PMC2935336/

Casla, S., Hojman, P., Márquez-Rodas, I., López-Tarruella, S., Jerez, Y., Barakat, R., & Martin, M. (2015). Running away from side effects: Physical exercise as a complementary intervention for breast cancer patients. *Clinical and translational oncology*, 17(3), 180-196. https://www.ncbi.nlm.nih.gov/pubmed/24894838

Courneya, K. S., Segal, R. J., McKenzie, D. C., Dong, H., Gelmon, K., Friedenreich, C. M., & Mackey, J. R. (2014). Effects of exercise during adjuvant chemotherapy on breast cancer outcomes. *Medicine & Science in Sports & Exercise, 46*(9), 1744-1751. https://www.ncbi.nlm.nih.gov/pubmed/24633595

Gray et. al., 2015. Cumulative use of strong anticholinergics and incident dementia: A prospective cohort study. *JAMA Internal Medicine, 175* (3). Retrieved from http://archinte.jamanetwork.com/article.aspx?articleid=2091745

Group, E. (2015). 6 Toxins that destroy your thyroid. *Global Healing Center*. Retrieved from http://www.globalhealingcenter.com/natural-health/6-toxins-that-destroy-your-thyroid/

Harvard Health, The Nutrition Source (2017). Alcohol: Balancing risks and benefits. Retrieved from https://www.hsph.harvard.edu/nutritionsource/alcohol-full-story/

Kunkler, P. E., Zhang, L., Pellman, J. J., Oxford, G. S., & Hurley, J. H. (2015). Sensitization of the trigeminovascular system following environmental irritant exposure. *Cephalalgia*, 0333102415574845. https://www.ncbi.nlm.nih.gov/pubmed/25724913

Martin, R. W., & Becker, C. (1993). Headaches from chemical exposures. *Headache: The Journal of Head and Face Pain, 33*(10), 555-559. https://www.ncbi.nlm.nih.gov/pubmed/?term=martin+chemical+exposure+headache

National Research Council. (1991). Review of the National Human Adipose Tissue Survey and selected program alternatives. https://www.ncbi.nlm.nih.gov/books/NBK234182/

Lavigne, É., Bélair, M. A., Do, M. T., Stieb, D. M., Hystad, P., van Donkelaar, A., ... & Brook, J. R. (2017). Maternal exposure to ambient air pollution and risk of early childhood cancers: A population-based study in Ontario, Canada. *Environment International*. https://www.ncbi.nlm.nih.gov/pubmed/28108116

Pedersen, M., Andersen, Z. J., Stafoggia, M., Weinmayr, G., Galassi, C., Sørensen, M., & Nagel, G. (2017). Ambient air pollution and primary liver cancer incidence in four European cohorts within the ESCAPE project. *Environmental Research, 154*, 226-233. https://www.ncbi.nlm.nih.gov/pubmed/28107740

Sherr, David. (2013). Environmental pollutants and the immune system. Physiscans For Social Responsibility. Written with Boston University School of Public Health. http://www.psr.org/Chapters/boston/resources/environmental-pollutants-and-the-immune-system.html?referrer=https://www.google.ca/

Tinker, B. (2016) Common over-the-counter drugs can hurt your brain. *CNN online*. Retrieved from http://www.cnn.com/2016/04/18/health/otc-anticholinergic-drugs-dementia/

Wolf, M. S., King, J., Jacobson, K., Di Francesco, L., Bailey, S. C., Mullen, R., & Parker, R. M. (2012). Risk of unintentional overdose with non-prescription acetaminophen products. *Journal of General Internal Medicine, 27*(12), 1587-1593. https://www.ncbi.nlm.nih.gov/pmc/articles/PMC3509295/

CHAPTER 17

The Holmes and Rahe stress scales: Understanding the impact of long-term stress. (n.d.). *Mind Tools*. Retrieved from https://www.mindtools.com/pages/article/newTCS_82.htm

Gillson, G., & Marsden, T. (2004). *You've hit menopause: Now what? 3 simple steps to restoring hormone balance*. Calgary: Blitzprint. Retrieved from http://rmalab.com/sites/default/files/files/YHMNW2ndEd(1).pdf

CHAPTER 18

Moorjani, Anita. (2012). *Dying to be me*. Carlsbad, CA: Hay House.

Tolle, Eckhardt. (1999). *The power of now*. Novato, CA: New World Library.

Inspiration. (n.d.). *Online Etymology Dictionary*. Retrieved from http://www.etymonline.com/index.php?term=inspiration

Northup, C. (2006). *Mother-daughter wisdom: Understanding the crucial link between mothers, daughters, and health*. New York: Random House.

Hay, Louise. (1984). *You can heal your life*. Carlsbad, CA: Hay House.

Chopra, D., Ford, D., Williamson, (2010). *The shadow effect: Illuminating the hidden power of your true self*. San Francisco: HarperOne.

Fenstemaker, S. (2012). What are shadow beliefs. *People-triggers*.

Retrieved from https://peopletriggers.wordpress.com/2012/05/21/what-are-shadow-beliefs/#respond

Levin, N. (2014). *Jump! And Your Life Will Appear*. Carlsbad, CA: Hay House.

Luna, A. (n.d.). What are your core beliefs and why are they so important to uncover? *Loner Wolf*. Retrieved from https://lonerwolf.com/core-beliefs/

Greenberger, D. & Padesky, C. (1995). *Mind over mood*. New York: The Guilford Press.

CHAPTER 19

Hall, Karyn D. (2014). *The emotionally sensitive person: Finding peace when your emotions overwhelm you*. Oakland, CA: New Harbinger Publications.

Aron, Elaine. (1996). *The highly sensitive person: How to thrive when the world overwhelms you*. New York: Broadway Books.

Holden, Robert. (2009). *Be happy!* Carlsbad, CA: Hay House.

Winfrey, O. (n.d.). Uncovering your shadow beliefs. *Oprah.com*. Retrieved from http://www.oprah.com/spirit/Uncovering-Your-Shadow-Beliefs

CHAPTER 20

Journal of Naturopathic Medicine

Tipping, Colin. (2009). *Radical forgiveness*. Boulder, CO: Sounds True, 2009.

Walsch, Neale. (1998). *Little soul and the sun*. Charlottesville, VA: Hampton Roads Publishing Company.

Williamson, Marianne. (1996). *A return to love*. San Francisco: HarperOne.

Hay, Louise. (1984). *You can heal your life*. Carlsbad, CA: Hay House.

Seligman, Martin. (2002). *Authentic happiness*. New York: Atria Paperback / Simon & Schuster Inc.

Peterson, Christopher. (2006). *A primer in positive psychology*. New York: Oxford University Press.

Kipp, M. (2013) Heart therapy with Mastin Kipp of TheDailyLove.com [Glimpserv].

Northrup, C. (1994). *Women's bodies, women's wisdom*. New York: Bantam Books.

Kate Northrup. [YouTube]. Retrieved from https://www.youtube.com/watch?v=vfZxdDort7o

Brach, T. (2014). *From fight-flight-freeze to attend-befriend: Conflict* (part 2). [YouTube]. Retrieved from https://www.youtube.com/watch?v=a25t4klaQDs

CHAPTER 21

World Health Organization (2001). Mental disorders affect in one in four. Retrieved from http://www.who.int/whr/2001/media_centre/press_release/en

Canadian Mental Health Association. Violence and mental health: Unpacking a complex issue. Retrieved from http://ontario.cmha.ca/public_policy/violence-and-mental-health-unpacking-a-complex-issue/#.vYq8xPlViko

Andreasen, N. (2014). Secrets of the creative brain. *The Atlantic,* July/August. Retrieved from http://www.theatlantic.com/features/archive/2014/06/secrets-of-the-creative-brain/372299

List of people with major depressive disorder Person Centred Care Chart CMHA. *Wikipedia*. Retrieved from https://en.wikipedia.org/wiki/List_of_people_with_major_depressive_disorder

CMHA Person Centered Care Chart

APPENDIX

Morley, Carol. (2010). *Delicious detox* for Green goddess; Blueberry buckwheat pancakes, Almond chicken, Asian asparagus, Flax baked chicken, Roasted beets and spinach salad, Berry-almond slam smoothie, Warm spicy sweet potato salad, Chickpea slaw, Fresh salad rolls and tangy almond dipping sauce. deliciousdetoxcookbook.com

Daniluk, Julie: *Meals that Heal Inflammation* for: Blueberry hemp smoothie; Crispy kale chips, Raw pad Thai, Cranberry quiona salad, Grain-free berry muffins, Ginger butternut soup, Lentil dip, Arugula rainbow salad, Kale salad

Curried chicken salad from www.foodnetwork.com/recipes/tyler-florence/curried-chicken-salad-sandwich-with-almonds-and-raisins-recipe.html

Vegan mayo from www.thekitchn.com/how-to-make-easy-vegan-mayonnaise-227726

Salmon with balsamic glaze from www.foodnetwork.ca/recipe/grilled-salmon-with-balsamiconion-glaze/9965/

Lentil vegetable soup adapted from www.glutenfreeliving.com/recipes/soupsstews/vegan-lentil-soup/

Cornmeal carrot muffins adapted from www.food.com/recipe/corn-carrot-muffins-190174

Ginger chicken stir fry from www.chatelaine.com/recipe/vegetables/ginger-chicken-stirfry-with-greens/

Banana nut butter spread from www.blenderbabes.com/lifestyle-diet/dairy-free/banananut-butter-spread-recipe/

Soba noodle veggie pot adapted from www.restlesspalate.com/asian-soba-noodles purple-cabbage/

Three-bean vegetarian chili from www.myrecipes.com/recipe/three-bean-vegetarian-chili

Apple and hazelnut muesli from www.theguardian.com/lifeandstyle/wordofmouth/2014/oct/23/how-to-make-perfect-bircher-muesli-recipe

No-noodle zucchini lasagna from www.allrecipes.com/recipe/172958/no-noodle-zucchinilasagna/

Crispy breakfast bars from www.vegetariantimes.com/recipe/crispy-breakfast-bars/

Shrimp in Thai green curry from www.thaikitchen.com/Recipes/Seafood/Green-Curry-Shrimp

Breakfast sausages adapted from www.healthylivinghowto.com/1/post/2012/07/say-goodbye-to-jimmy-dean.html

Challem, Jack. (2010). *The inflammation syndrome: Your nutrition plan for great health, weight loss, and pain-free living* for: Wonderful whatever salad

Vegetarian chili with avocado salsa from www.myrecipes.com/recipe/quickvegetarian-chili-with-avocado-salsa

Sesame-seed-crusted salmon burgers from *Health* magazine www.health.com/health/recipe/0,,10000001990042,00.html

Edamame and bean salad with shrimp and fresh salsa from www.myrecipes.com/recipe/edamame-bean-salad-with-shrimp-fresh-salsa

Spaghetti squash and black bean tacos adapted from Perelman, Deb. (2012). *The Smitten Kitchen Cookbook*: https://blueberriesandbasil.wordpress.com/2015/09/24/smitten-kitchens-spaghetti-squash-tacos-with-black-beans-and-queso-fresco/

Stewed kale and lentils from www.canadianliving.com/food/quick-and-easy/recipe/stewed-kale-and-lentils

Denby, Nigel. (2007). GL *Cookbook and Diet Plan* for: Warm oat and apple bowl

Garden bean soup adapted from www.myrecipes.com/recipe/curriedlentil-chickpea-stew

Pumpkin-seed-crusted halibut from www.epicurious.com/recipes/food/views/grilled-halibut-with-coriander-pepita-butter 35333

Ready to Reclaim Your Mental Health?
Join My Next Moving Beyond Coaching Group!

MOVING BEYOND COACHING is an instructional program that addresses the physical, mental, emotional and spiritual aspects of mental health. I have a course for health care providers and for individuals who want support additional to what their current health care provider is offering.

I am here to ensure that you create meaningful and lasting change. Let me support you in taking action to free yourself from the mental prison you might be trapped inside. Take the first step from moving from where you are to where you desire to be right now! To express my appreciation and gratitude to you for purchasing this book, I am gifting you a savings on an upcoming Moving Beyond Coaching Program. Please visit naturalterrain.com/moving-beyond-coaching-program/ and enter the code MENTALHEALTH to receive your C$100 discount.

Due to the nature of this work, I only work with a handful of people one-on-one at a time. If you feel private care is what you need, please reach out to me via my website and I can make suggestions for you.

What others have to say about the Moving Beyond Coaching Program:

The "Moving Beyond" course is a unique learning experience. Not only will you learn relevant, practical and tangible clinical information to utilize with patients right away, you will also learn the importance of "physician, heal thyself," which can often be missing in other professional educational courses, allowing you to put into practice what you're learning.

Dr. Chris draws upon her own personal and professional experiences in the area of mental health in an engaging and dynamic way, sharing personal and clinical examples, concepts, techniques and tools learned from various sources providing a foundation for acquiring knowledge and skills for an effective and integrated approach in serving others. The small group setting was intimate, supportive and relaxed, with invitation to share, discuss or just listen. I enjoyed my experience and I'm sure you will enjoy it as well.

DR. H., COURSE PARTICIPANT

This course is amazing! I have learned so much and Dr. Chris is such a great teacher :)
DR. S., COURSE PARTICIPANT

Your material is awesome and you're a great presenter. THANK YOU!! As an ND, I always learn something each week—new and refreshing information. Love the physiology charts and pathways with cofactors. I especially enjoy your analogies because these are always helpful to share with patients to help them understand their current challenges in everyday language. Your content and knowledge level in this area is all encompassing and well laid out/researched and will help a ton of people out there. You're a champion!!! THANK YOU!
DR. N., COURSE PARTICIPANT

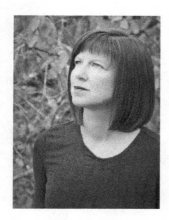

DR. CHRISTINA BJORNDAL, B. Comm, ND, graduated from the University of British Columbia in 1990 with a Bachelor of Commerce Degree with honours. She was valedictorian of her graduating class. She completed her doctorate in naturopathic medicine from the Canadian College of Naturopathic Medicine in 2005. She is one of the only licensed NDs in Canada who is considered an authority in the treatment of mental illnesses such as depression, anxiety, bipolar disorders, eating disorders, ADD/ADHD, OCD and schizo-affective disorders. A gifted speaker and writer, she has shared her personal story and philosophy of wellness with audiences across North America. Dr. Chris has helped many patients navigate through labels and stigma toward physical, mental, emotional and spiritual well-being. Having overcome many challenges in the sphere of mental health, Dr. Chris is especially exceptional about sharing in her motivational speeches how to overcome barriers in life and encouraging others to achieve their full potential. She loves her work and balances it with a full, active lifestyle with her husband and son. To learn more about her books, courses and retreat, please visit: naturalterrain.com. If you would like Dr. Chris to speak at an event, please contact her at admin@naturalterrain.com or call 587-521-3595.

CPSIA information can be obtained
at www.ICGtesting.com
Printed in the USA
BVHW091022150922
647127BV00001B/33